Mosby's

PHYSICAL EXAMINATION HANDBOOK

Henry M. Seidel, MD
Professor Emeritus of Pediatrics
The Johns Hopkins University School of Medicine
Baltimore, Maryland

Jane W. Ball, RN, DrPH, CPNP, NAP
Executive Director
National Resource Center
Children's National Medical Center
Washington, DC

Joyce E. Dains, DrPH, JD, RN, FNP, BC, NAP
Manager
Professional Education for Prevention and Early Detection
The University of Texas M.D. Anderson Cancer Center
Houston, Texas

G. William Benedict, MD, PhD
Assistant Professor, Medicine
The Johns Hopkins University School of Medicine
Baltimore, Maryland

MOSBY
ELSEVIER

MOSBY
ELSEVIER

11830 Westline Industrial Drive
St. Louis, Missouri 63146

MOSBY'S PHYSICAL EXAMINATION HANDBOOK,
SIXTH EDITION   ISBN-13: 978-0-323-03231-5
                                 ISBN-10: 0-323-03231-1

ISBN-13: 978-0-323-03231-5
ISBN-10: 0-323-03231-1

Executive Publisher: Robin Carter
Developmental Editor: Deanna Davis
Publishing Services Manager: Deborah L. Vogel
Project Manager: Katherine Hinkebein
Cover and Text Designer: Jyotika Shroff

Printed in the United States of America

Last digit is the print number: 9 8 7 6 5 4 3 2 1

PREFACE

Mosby's Physical Examination Handbook, Sixth Edition, is a portable clinical reference on physical examination suitable for students of nursing, medicine, chiropractic, and other allied health disciplines, as well as for practicing health care providers. It offers brief descriptions of examination techniques and guidelines on how the examination should proceed, step by step. This handbook is intended to be an aid to review and recall of the procedures of physical examination. It cannot, because of its brevity, describe the specific techniques of history taking by organ system.

The handbook begins with an outline of what information should be obtained for the patient's medical history and review of systems. Subsequent chapters for each of the body systems list equipment needed to perform the examination and present the techniques to be used. Expected and unexpected findings follow the description of each technique, presented in distinctive color type for easy recognition. Numerous illustrations interspersed throughout the text reinforce techniques and possible findings.

Each chapter offers Aids to Differential Diagnosis and also provides Sample Documentation, which in this edition has been focused on a specific complaint to illustrate good documentation practice. Pediatric Variations are also highlighted in each body systems chapter.

As in previous editions, separate chapters give an overview of the entire examination for all adults; for healthy females; and for infants, children, and adolescents. The final chapter gives guidelines for reporting and recording findings.

New to this edition is an expanded appendix of special histories. This appendix now includes the HEEADSSS screening tool for adolescents, along with such other useful tools as the TACE questionnaire (for detecting risk drinking), the RAFFT questionnaire (for detecting substance abuse in adolescents), and several additional special histories.

Henry M. Seidel
Jane W. Ball
Joyce E. Dains
G. William Benedict

CONTENTS

THE HISTORY

TAKING THE HISTORY

The following outline of a patient history should be viewed not as a rigid structure but as a general guideline. Since you are beginning your relationship with the patient at this point, pay attention to this relationship as well as to the information you seek in the history. Be friendly and show respect for the patient. Choose a comfortable setting and help the patient get settled. Maintain eye contact and use a conversational tone. Begin by introducing yourself and explaining your role. Help the patient understand why you are taking the history and how it will be used. Once the history proceeds, explore positive responses with additional questions: where, when, what, how, and why. Be sensitive to the patient's emotions at all times. Avoid confrontation and asking leading questions.

CHIEF COMPLAINT

Problem or symptom: Reason for visit
Duration of problem
Patient information: Age, sex, marital status, previous hospital admissions; occupation
Other complaints: Secondary issues, fears, concerns, what made patient seek care
Always consider why this particular problem may be affecting this particular patient at this time. Why did this patient succumb to a risk or an exposure when others similarly exposed did not?

PRESENT PROBLEM

Chronologic ordering: Sequence of events patient has experienced
State of health just before onset of present problem
Complete description of first symptom: Time and date of onset, location, movement
Possible exposure to infection or toxic agents

If symptoms are intermittent, describe typical attack: Onset, duration, symptoms, variations, inciting factors, exacerbating factors, relieving factors

Impact of illness: On lifestyle, on ability to function; limitations imposed by illness

"Stability" of problem: Intensity, variations, improvement, worsening, staying same

Immediate reason for seeking attention, particularly for long-standing problem

Review of appropriate system when there is a conspicuous disturbance of a particular organ or system

Medications: Current and recent, dosage of prescriptions, home remedies, nonprescription medications

Review of chronology of events for each problem: Patient's confirmations and corrections

MEDICAL HISTORY

General health and strength

Childhood illnesses: Measles, mumps, whooping cough, chicken-pox, smallpox, scarlet fever, acute rheumatic fever, diphtheria, poliomyelitis

Major adult illnesses: Tuberculosis (TB), hepatitis, diabetes, hypertension, myocardial infarction, tropical or parasitic diseases, other infections, any nonsurgical hospital admissions

Immunizations: Poliomyelitis, diphtheria, pertussis, tetanus toxoid, influenza, *Haemophilus influenzae* B, pneumococcal, cholera, typhus, typhoid, bacille Calmette-Guérin (BCG), hepatitis B virus (HBV), last purified protein derivative (PPD) or other skin tests; unusual reactions to immunizations; tetanus or other antitoxin made with horse serum

Surgery: Dates, hospital, diagnosis, complications

Serious injuries: Resulting disability (document fully for injuries with possible legal implications)

Limitation of ability to function as desired as a result of past events

Medications: Past, current, recent medications; dosage of prescription; home remedies and nonprescription medications, particularly complementary and alternative therapies

Allergies: Especially to medications but also to environmental allergens and foods

Transfusions: Reactions, date, number of units transfused

Emotional status: Mood disorders, psychiatric treatment

Children: Birth, developmental milestones, childhood diseases, immunizations

FAMILY HISTORY

The genetic basis for a patient's response to risk or exposure may determine whether the patient becomes ill when others do not.

Relatives with similar illness

Immediate family: Ethnicity, health, cause of and age at death

History of disease: Heart disease, high blood pressure, hypercholesterolemia, cancer, TB, stroke, epilepsy, diabetes, gout, kidney disease, thyroid disease, asthma and other allergic states, forms of arthritis, blood diseases, sexually transmitted diseases, other familial diseases

Spouse and children: Age, health

Hereditary disease: History of grandparents, aunts, uncles, siblings, cousins; consanguinity

PERSONAL AND SOCIAL HISTORY

Personal status: Birthplace, where raised, home environment; parental divorce or separation, socioeconomic class, cultural background, education, position in family, marital status, general life satisfaction, hobbies and interests, sources of stress and strain

Habits: Nutrition and diet; regularity and patterns of eating and sleeping; exercise: quantity and type; quantity of coffee, tea, tobacco, alcohol; illicit drug use: frequency, type, amount; breast or testicular self-examination

Sexual history: Concerns with sexual feelings and performance, frequency of intercourse, ability to achieve orgasm, number and gender of partners

Home conditions: Housing, economic condition, type of health insurance if any, pets and their health

Occupation: Description of usual work and present work if different; list of job changes; work conditions and hours; physical and mental strain; duration of employment; present and past exposure to heat and cold, industrial toxins (especially lead, arsenic, chromium, asbestos, beryllium, poisonous gases, benzene, and polyvinyl chloride or other carcinogens and teratogens); any protective devices required, for example, goggles or masks

Environment: Travel and other exposure to contagious diseases, residence in tropics, water and milk supply, other sources of infection if applicable

Military record: Dates and geographic area of assignments

Complementary and alternative health and medical systems: History and current use

Religious preference: Religious proscriptions concerning medical care

Cost of care: Resources available to patient, financial worries, candid discussion of issues

REVIEW OF SYSTEMS

It is unlikely that all questions in each system will be asked on every occasion. The following questions are among those that should be asked, particularly at a first interview.

General constitutional symptoms: Fever, chills, malaise, fatigability, night sweats, weight (average, preferred, present, change)

Skin, hair, nails: Rash or eruption, itching, pigmentation or texture change, excessive sweating, abnormal nail or hair growth

Head and neck:

> General: Frequent or unusual headaches, their location, dizziness, syncope, severe head injuries, periods of loss of consciousness (momentary or prolonged)
>
> Eyes: Visual acuity, blurring, diplopia, photophobia, pain, recent change in appearance or vision, glaucoma, use of eyedrops or other eye medications, history of trauma or familial eye disease
>
> Ears: Hearing loss, pain, discharge, tinnitus, vertigo
>
> Nose: Sense of smell, frequency of colds, obstruction, epistaxis, postnasal discharge, sinus pain
>
> Throat and mouth: Hoarseness or change in voice, frequent sore throats, bleeding or swelling of gums, recent tooth abscesses or extractions, soreness of tongue or buccal mucosa, ulcers, disturbance of taste

Lymph nodes: Enlargement, tenderness, suppuration

Chest and lungs: Pain related to respiration, dyspnea, cyanosis, wheezing, cough, sputum (character and quantity), hemoptysis, night sweats, exposure to TB, date and result of last chest x-ray examination

Breasts: Pain, tenderness, discharge, lumps, galactorrhea, mammograms (screening or diagnostic), frequency of self-examination

Heart and blood vessels: Chest pain or distress, precipitating causes, timing and duration, character, relieving factors, palpitations, dyspnea, orthopnea (number of pillows needed), edema, claudication, hypertension, previous myocardial infarction, estimate of exercise tolerance, past electrocardiogram (ECG) or other cardiac tests

Peripheral vasculature: Claudication (frequency, severity), tendency to bruise or bleed, thromboses, thrombophlebitis

Hematologic: Any known abnormality of blood cells, transfusions

Gastrointestinal: Appetite, digestion, intolerance of any class of foods, dysphagia, heartburn, nausea, vomiting, hematemesis; regularity of bowels, constipation, diarrhea, change in stool color or contents (clay colored, tarry, fresh blood, mucus, undigested food), flatulence, hemorrhoids; hepatitis, jaundice, dark urine; history of ulcer, gallstones, polyps, tumor; previous x-ray examinations (where, when, findings)

Diet: Appetite, likes and dislikes, restrictions (e.g., because of religion, allergy, or other disease), vitamins and other supplements, use of caffeine-containing beverages (e.g., coffee, tea, cola), an hour-by-hour detailing of food and liquid intake—sometimes a written diary covering several days of intake may be necessary

Endocrine: Thyroid enlargement or tenderness, heat or cold intolerance, unexplained weight change, diabetes, polydipsia, polyuria, changes in facial or body hair, increased hat and glove size, skin striae

Females:

Menses: Onset, regularity, duration and amount of flow, dysmenorrhea, date of last period (LMP), intermenstrual discharge or bleeding, itching, date of last Pap smear, age at menopause, libido, frequency of intercourse, sexual difficulties, infertility

Pregnancies: Number, living children, multiple births, miscarriages, abortions, duration of pregnancies, type of delivery for each, any complications during any pregnancy or postpartum period or with neonate, use of oral or other contraceptives, difficulty in getting pregnant

Males: Puberty onset, difficulty with erections, emissions, testicular pain, libido, infertility

Genitourinary: Dysuria, flank or suprapubic pain, urgency, frequency, nocturia, hematuria, polyuria, hesitancy, dribbling, loss in force of stream, passage of stone, edema of face, stress incontinence, hernias, sexually transmitted disease (inquire type and symptoms and results of serologic test for syphilis [STS], if known)

Musculoskeletal: Joint stiffness, pain, restriction of motion, swelling, redness, heat, bony deformity

Neurologic: Syncope, seizures, weakness or paralysis, abnormalities of sensation or coordination, tremors, loss of memory

Psychiatric: Depression, mood changes, difficulty concentrating, nervousness, tension, suicidal thoughts, irritability, sleep disturbances

CONCLUDING QUESTIONS

In conclusion, ask:

Is there anything else that you think would be important for me to know?

If there are several problems: Which concerns you the most?

If the history is vague, complicated, or contradictory: What do you think is the matter with you, or, what worries you the most?

TAKING THE HISTORY

These are only guidelines; you are free to modify and add as the needs of your patients and your judgment dictate.

CHIEF COMPLAINT

A parent or other responsible adult will generally be the major resource. When age permits, however, child should be involved as much as possible. Remember that every chief complaint has the potential of an underlying concern. What really led to the visit to you? Was it just the sore throat?

RELIABILITY

Note relationship to patient of person who is the resource for history, and record your impression of the competence of that person as a historian.

PRESENT PROBLEM

Be sure to give a clear chronologic sequence to the story.

MEDICAL HISTORY

In general, the age of the patient and/or the nature of the problem will guide your approach to the history. Clearly, in a continuing relationship much of what is to be known will already have been recorded. Certainly, different aspects of the history require varying emphasis depending on the nature of the immediate problem. There are specifics that will command attention.

Pregnancy/mother's health:
    Infectious disease; give approximate gestational month
    Weight gain/edema
    Hypertension
    Proteinuria
    Bleeding; approximate time
    Eclampsia, threat of eclampsia
    Special or unusual diet or dietary practices
    Medications (hormones, vitamins)

Quality of fetal movements, time of onset
Radiation exposure
Prenatal care/consistency
Birth and perinatal experience:
Duration of pregnancy
Delivery site
Labor: Spontaneous/induced, duration, anesthesia, complications
Delivery: Presentation; forceps/spontaneous; complications
Condition at birth: Time of onset of cry; Apgar scores, if available
Birth weight and, if available, length and head circumference
Neonatal period:
Hospital experience: Length of stay, feeding experience, oxygen needs, vigor, color (jaundice, cyanosis), cry. Did baby go home with mother?
First month of life: Color (jaundice), feeding, vigor, any suggestion of illness or untoward event
Feeding:
Bottle or breast: Any changes and why; type of formula, amounts offered/taken, feeding frequency; weight gain
Present diet and appetite: Introduction of solids, current routine and frequency, age weaned from bottle or breast, daily intake of milk, food preferences, ability to feed self; elaborate on any feeding problems

DEVELOPMENT

Guidelines suggested in Chapter 21, Age-Specific Examination: Infants, Children, and Adolescents, are complementary to the milestones listed below. Those included here are commonly used, often remembered, and often recorded in "baby books." Photographs may also occasionally be of some help. NOTE: it is important to define the growth and developmental status of each child regardless of the particular complaint. That status will inform your understanding of the child, and of the particular problem, and will facilitate the institution of a management plan.
Age when:
Held head erect while held in sitting position
Sat alone, unsupported
Walked alone
Talked in sentences
Toilet trained

School: Grade, performance, learning and social problems

Dentition: Ages for first teeth, loss of deciduous teeth, first permanent teeth

Growth: Height and weight at different ages, changes in rate of growth or weight gain or loss

Sexual: Present status (e.g., in female, time of breast development, nipples, pubic hair, description of menses; in males, development of pubic hair, voice change, acne, emissions). Follow Tanner guides.

Growth: Height and weight at different ages, changes in rate of growth or weight gain or loss

Sexual: Present status (e.g., in female, time of breast development, nipples, pubic hair, description of menses; in males, development of pubic hair, voice change, acne, emissions). Follow Tanner guides.

FAMILY HISTORY

Maternal gestational history: All pregnancies with status of each, including date, age, cause of death of all deceased siblings, and dates and duration of pregnancy in the case of miscarriages; mother's health during pregnancy

Age of parents at birth of patient

Are parents related to each other in any way?

PERSONAL AND SOCIAL HISTORY

Personal status:
- School adjustment
- Nail biting
- Thumb sucking
- Breath holding
- Temper tantrums
- Pica
- Tics
- Rituals

Home conditions:
- Parental occupation(s)
- Principal caretaker(s) of patient
- Food preparation, routine, family preferences (e.g., vegetarianism), who does preparing
- Adequacy of clothing

Dependency on relief or social agencies
Number of persons and rooms in house or apartment
Sleeping routines and sleeping arrangements for child

REVIEW OF SYSTEMS (SOME SUGGESTED ADDITIONAL QUESTIONS OR PARTICULAR CONCERNS)

Ears: Otitis media (frequency, laterality)
Nose: Snoring, mouth breathing
Teeth: Dental care
Genitourinary: Nature of urinary stream, forceful or a dribble
Skin, hair, nails: Eczema or seborrhea

MENTAL STATUS

EQUIPMENT

- Familiar objects (coins, keys, paper clips)
- Paper and pencil

EXAMINATION

Perform the mental status examination throughout the patient interaction. Focus on the individual's strengths and capabilities for executive functioning (motivation, initiative, goal formation, planning and performing work or activities, self-monitoring, and integrating feedback from various sources to refine or redirect energy). Interview a family member or friend if you have any concerns about the patient's responses or behaviors.

Use a mental status screening examination for health visits when no cognitive, emotional, or behavior problems are apparent. Information is generally observed during the history in the following areas:

Appearance and behavior
    Grooming
    Emotional status
    Body language

Cognitive abilities
    State of consciousness
    Memory
    Attention span
    Judgment

Emotional stability
    Mood and feelings
    Thought process and content

Speech and language
    Voice quality
    Articulation
    Comprehension
    Coherence
    Ability to communicate

TECHNIQUE   **FINDINGS**

MENTAL STATUS AND SPEECH PATTERNS

Observe physical appearance and behavior

■ *Grooming*

UNEXPECTED: Poor hygiene; lack of concern with appearance; or inappropriate dress for season, gender, or occasion in previously well-groomed patient.

■ *Emotional status*

EXPECTED: Patient expressing concern with visit that is appropriate for emotional content of topics discussed.

UNEXPECTED: Behavior conveying carelessness, indifference, inability to sense emotions in others, loss of sympathetic reactions, unusual docility, rage reactions, agitation, or excessive irritability.

■ *Body language*

EXPECTED: Erect posture and eye contact (if culturally appropriate).

UNEXPECTED: Slumped posture, lack of facial expression, inappropriate affect, excessively energetic movements, or constantly watchful eyes.

Investigate cognitive abilities

■ *Six-Item Cognitive Impairment Test*
Use this test to assess cognition (see p. 12).

EXPECTED: Score less than 10.

UNEXPECTED: Score between 10 and 28.

Six-Item Cognitive Impairment Test

Item	Maximum Error	Score	Weight	Final Item Score
1. What *year* is it now?	1		4	
2. What *month* is it now?	1		3	
Memory phrase: Repeat this phrase after me: "*John Brown, 42 Market Street, Chicago*"				
3. About what time is it now? (within an hour)	1		3	
4. Count backwards 20 to 1	2		2	
5. Say the months in reverse order	2		2	
6. Repeat the memory phrase	5		2	

The Six-Item Cognitive Impairment Test. Assign 0 for a correct score, and 1 for each incorrect score up to the maximum number of errors permitted. Multiply the item score by the item weight to obtain the final item score. The maximum total score possible is 28. A score of 10 or higher is significant and should be referred. *From Brooke, Bullock, 1999.*

TECHNIQUE

- *Mini-Mental State Examination (MMSE)** Use this examination to quantify cognitive function or document changes.

- *State of consciousness*

- *Set Test* Use this test to evaluate mental status as a whole (motivation, alertness, concentration, short-term memory, problem solving). Ask patient to name

FINDINGS

EXPECTED: Score of 21 to 30.
UNEXPECTED: Score of 20 or less.

EXPECTED: Oriented to time, place, and person, and able to appropriately respond to questions and environmental stimuli.
UNEXPECTED: Disoriented to time, place, or person. Verbal response is confused, incoherent, or inappropriate, or there is no verbal response.

EXPECTED: Able to categorize, count, remember items listed. Score of 25 or more points.
UNEXPECTED: Score less than 15 points. Check for

---

*MMSE can be obtained from Psychological Assessment Resources, Inc., PO Box 998, Odessa, FL 33556; phone: 1-800-331-8378; www.minimental.com.

TECHNIQUE	**FINDINGS**
10 items in each of 4 groups: fruit, animals, colors, town/cities. Give each item 1 point for a maximum of 40 points.	mental changes or cultural, educational, or social factors when score is 15 to 24.
■ *Analogies* Ask patient to describe analogies, first simple, then more complex: • What is similar about peaches and lemons, oceans and lakes, pencil and typewriter? • An engine is to an airplane as an oar is to a _____? • What is different about a magazine and a telephone book, or a bush and a tree?	**EXPECTED:** Correct responses when patient has average intelligence. **UNEXPECTED:** Unable to describe similarities or differences.
■ *Abstract reasoning* Ask patient to explain meaning of fable, proverb, or metaphor: • A stitch in time saves nine. • A bird in the hand is worth two in the bush. • A rolling stone gathers no moss.	**EXPECTED:** Adequate interpretation when patient has average intelligence **UNEXPECTED:** Unable to give adequate explanation.
■ *Arithmetic calculations* Ask patient to perform simple calculations without paper and pencil: • $50 - 7, - 7, - 7$, etc., until answer is 8. • $50 + 8, + 8, + 8$, etc., until answer is 98.	**UNEXPECTED:** Unable to complete with few errors within a minute.
■ *Writing ability* Ask patient to write name and address or a phrase you dictate (or draw simple figures—triangle, circle, square, flower, house— if unable to write).	**UNEXPECTED:** Omission or addition of letters, syllables, or words; mirror writing; or uncoordinated writing (or drawing for patients unable to write).
■ *Execution of motor skills* Ask patient to do a motor task such as combing hair or putting on lipstick.	**UNEXPECTED:** Unable to complete a task.

TECHNIQUE	FINDINGS

■ *Memory*
Immediate recall or new learning: Ask patient to listen to, then repeat, a sentence or series of numbers (five to eight numbers forward, four to six numbers backward).
Recent memory: Show patient four or five objects or give visually impaired patient four unrelated words with distinct sounds to remember (carpet, iris, bench, fortune). Say you will ask about them later. In 10 minutes, ask patient to list objects.
Remote memory: Ask patient about verifiable past events (e.g., mother's maiden name, name of high school).

EXPECTED: *Immediate recall:* Able to repeat sentence or numbers.
Recent memory: Able to remember test objects.
Remote memory: Able to recall verifiable past events.
UNEXPECTED: Impaired memory. Loss of immediate and recent memory with retention of remote memory.

■ *Attention span*
Ask patient to follow a series of short commands (e.g., take off all clothes, put on patient gown, sit on examining table).

EXPECTED: Responds to directions appropriately.
UNEXPECTED: Easy distraction or confusion, negativism.

■ *Judgment*
Explore:
• How patient meets social and family obligations, patient's future plans.
• Patient's solutions to hypothetical situations (e.g., found stamped envelope or was stopped for running red light).

EXPECTED: Able to evaluate situation and provide appropriate response; managing business affairs appropriately.
UNEXPECTED: Response indicating hazardous behavior or inappropriate action.

Evaluate emotional stability

■ *Mood and feelings*
Ask patient how he or she feels, whether feelings are a problem in daily life, and whether he or she has particularly difficult times or experiences.

EXPECTED: Appropriate feelings for the situation.
UNEXPECTED:
Unresponsiveness, hopelessness, agitation, aggression, anger, euphoria,

TECHNIQUE	FINDINGS

irritability, or wide mood swings.

■ *Geriatric Depression Scale*
Use this test to assess for possible depression in older adults (see below).

EXPECTED: Score of 5 or less.

UNEXPECTED: Score greater than 5.

■ *Thought process and content*
• Ask patient about obsessive thoughts relating to making decisions, fears, or guilt.
• Ask patient about the need to compulsively repeat actions, check, and recheck (or observe the patient's actions).
• Observe sequence, logic, coherence, and relevance of topics.
• Does patient have delusions?

EXPECTED: Patient's thought processes can be followed, and expressed ideas are logical and goal directed.

UNEXPECTED: Illogical or unrealistic thought process, blocking, or disturbance in stream of thought. Obsessive thought content, compulsive behavior, phobias, anxieties that interfere with daily life or are disabling. Delusions.

Ask the patient to choose the best answer for how he or she felt over the previous week.

1. Are you basically satisfied with your life?	YES / NO
2. Have you dropped many of your activities and interests?	YES / NO
3. Do you feel that your life is empty?	YES / NO
4. Do you often get bored?	YES / NO
5. Are you in good spirits most of the time?	YES / NO
6. Are you afraid that something bad is going to happen to you?	YES / NO
7. Do you feel happy most of the time?	YES / NO
8. Do you feel helpless?	YES / NO
9. Do you prefer to stay at home, rather than going out and doing new things?	YES / NO
10. Do you feel you have more problems with memory than most?	YES / NO
11. Do you think it is wonderful to be alive now?	YES / NO
12. Do you feel pretty worthless the way you are now?	YES / NO
13. Do you feel full of energy?	YES / NO
14. Do you feel that your situation is hopeless?	YES / NO
15. Do you think most people are better off than you are?	YES / NO

Correct responses are the following:
  Yes for questions 2, 3, 4, 6, 8, 9, 10, 12, 14, and 15.
  No for questions 1, 5, 7, 11, and 13.
Give one point for each correct answer. A score greater than five suggests depression.

Geriatric Depression Scale. *From Sheikh, Yesavage, 1986.*

TECHNIQUE	**FINDINGS**

■ *Perceptual distortions and hallucinations*
Ask patient about any sensations not believed to be caused by external stimuli. Find out when these experiences occur.

UNEXPECTED: Sensory hallucinations—hears voices, sees vivid images or shadowy figures, smells offensive odors, feels worms crawling on skin.

Observe speech and language

■ *Voice quality*

EXPECTED: Uses inflections, speaks clearly and strongly, is able to increase voice volume and pitch.
UNEXPECTED: Difficulty or discomfort making laryngeal speech sounds or varying volume, quality, or pitch of speech.

■ *Articulation*

EXPECTED: Proper pronunciation, fluent, rhythmic; easily expresses thoughts.
UNEXPECTED: Imperfect pronunciation, difficulty articulating single speech sound, rapid-fire delivery, or speech with hesitancy, stuttering, repetitions, or slow utterances.

■ *Comprehension*

EXPECTED: Able to follow simple instructions.

■ *Coherence*

EXPECTED: Able to clearly convey intentions or perceptions.
UNEXPECTED: Circumlocutions, perseveration, flight of ideas or loosening of associations between thoughts, gibberish, neologisms, clang association, echolalia, or unusual sounds.

■ *Ability to communicate*

UNEXPECTED: Hesitations, omissions, inappropriate word substitutions, circumlocutions, neologisms, disturbance of rhythm or words in sequence or other signs of aphasia.

AIDS TO DIFFERENTIAL DIAGNOSIS

ABNORMALITY	DESCRIPTION
Dementia	Insidious onset; depressed, apathetic mood persists. Rambling or incoherent speech. Memory, judgment, thought patterns, calculations impaired. Progressive condition.
Delirium	Sudden onset; condition lasts for hours or days. Mood and affect include rapid mood swings, fear, suspicion. Rambling and irrelevant conversation, illogical flow of ideas, and hallucinations are common. Sleep-wake cycle may be disturbed.
Dementia of Alzheimer's type	Subtle, insidious onset—generally with early memory loss, impaired ability to learn new information, or disturbance in executive functioning—leading to profound disintegration of personality and complete disorientation. Varied duration and rate of progression.
Depression	Altered mood and affect with extreme sadness, anxiety, irritability. Lack of motivation, lethargic or restless, and agitated. Poor concentration.
Anxiety disorder	Marked anxiety or fear that interferes with personal, social, occupational functioning. Panic attacks with symptoms such as palpitations, tachycardia, sweating, shaking, trembling, choking, chest pain, abdominal distress, dizziness, faintness.
Mental retardation	Subaverage intellectual functioning, deficits in adaptive behavior, inability to discriminate among stimuli, impaired short-term memory, lack of motivation.

PEDIATRIC VARIATIONS

EXAMINATION

TECHNIQUE	FINDINGS

MENTAL STATUS

TECHNIQUE	FINDINGS
Use parent's impressions of infant's responsiveness to guide your assessment	**EXPECTED:** Infant responds appropriately to parent's voice—is attentive, comforts easily. Child follows simple directions, performs age-appropriate skills (see Chapter 17). **UNEXPECTED:** Nonresponsive, inconsolable, combative, lethargic.

AIDS TO DIFFERENTIAL DIAGNOSIS

ABNORMALITY	DESCRIPTION
Autistic disorder	Developmental disorder with odd repetitive behaviors, preoccupation with objects, an aversion to touch, delayed language or echolalia. Motor development may progress as expected.
Attention deficit hyperactivity disorder	Developmentally inappropriate inattention, hyperactivity, impulsivity, temper bursts, labile moods.

SAMPLE DOCUMENTATION

Subjective. A 16-year-old male fell playing basketball and struck the back of his head on a wooden floor. No loss of consciousness, got up and walked immediately, was dazed and confused for a few moments, has a headache.

Objective. Oriented to time, place, person. Reasoning and arithmetic calculation abilities intact. Immediate, recent, and remote memory intact. Appropriate mood and feeling expressed. Speech clearly and smoothly enunciated. Comprehends directions.

NUTRITION AND GROWTH AND MEASUREMENT

EQUIPMENT

- Tape measure with millimeter markings
- Devices for measuring weight and height
- Calculator
- Skinfold caliper

EXAMINATION

TECHNIQUE   **FINDINGS**

ANTHROPOMETRICS

Measure height and weight

- *Estimate desirable body weight (DBW)*
  Add 10% for large frame; subtract 10% for small frame.

  EXPECTED: *Women:* 100 pounds for first 5 feet, plus 5 pounds for each inch thereafter. *Men:* 106 pounds for first 5 feet, plus 6 pounds for each inch thereafter.

  Use growth charts for pediatric patients (pp. 290-300).

  EXPECTED: Child is following a growth curve pattern for height and weight. Height and weight are approximately same percentiles.

- *Calculate percent weight change*

  $$\left(\frac{\text{Usual weight} - \text{Current weight}}{\text{Usual weight}}\right) \times 100$$

  UNEXPECTED: Weight loss that equals or exceeds 1% to 2% in 1 week, 5% in 1 month, 7.5% in 3 months, 10% in 6 months.

TECHNIQUE	**FINDINGS**

■ *Calculate body mass index (BMI) (kg/m²)*

$$\left(\frac{\text{Weight in pounds} \times 703}{\text{Height in inches}} \right) \div \text{Height in inches}$$

or

see nomogram below. Also, see an interactive BMI calculator on the textbook Companion CD.

EXPECTED: 18.5 to 24.9 for both men and women.

UNEXPECTED: BMI above 25-29.9 is classified as *overweight*. BMI above 30.0 corresponds with obesity class I.

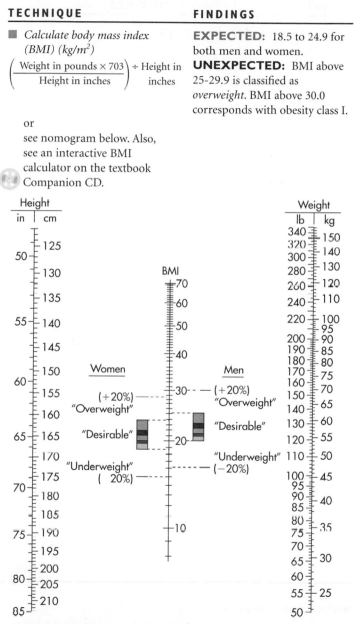

Nomogram for body mass index (kg/m²). Weight/height² is read from the central scale. The ranges suggested as "desirable" are from life insurance data.
From Thomas AE et al, 1976.

TECHNIQUE	FINDINGS

Calculate waist-to-hip circumference ratio

Using tape measure with millimeter markings, measure waist at or 1 cm above umbilical midline. Then measure hip at level of superior iliac crest. Divide waist circumference by hip circumference to obtain the ratio.

EXPECTED: Ratio less than 0.9 in men and 0.8 in women. **UNEXPECTED:** Ratios over 0.9 in men and 0.8 in women indicate increased central fat distribution and increased risk of disease.

DETERMINE DIET ADEQUACY

24-hour diet recall
Food diary

Use the MyPyramid guide at www.mypyramid.gov to track and analyze individual eating patterns and to generate a dietary plan based on age, gender, and physical activity level.

DETERMINE NUTRITIONAL ADEQUACY

Calculate estimates for energy needs

Use actual weight for healthy adults.
Use adjusted weight for obese patients.

Adjusted weight = [(Actual body weight − DBW) × 25%] + DBW

Calories	Kcal/kg
Weight loss	25
Weight maintenance	30
Weight gain	35
Hypermetabolic/ malnourished	35-50

Estimate fat intake

25% to 35% of the daily calories consumed should come from fat, with a distribution of
<7% saturated fat,
<10% polyunsaturated fat, and the rest in monounsaturated fat.

Estimate protein intake

An average of 0.8 g per kilogram body weight is sufficient to meet needs. Approximately 25% of

TECHNIQUE	FINDINGS
	daily calories consumed should come from protein.
Estimate carbohydrate intake	
	50% to 60% of the total calories consumed should come from carbohydrates, which should be predominately complex carbohydrates including grains, fruits, and vegetables.
Estimate fiber intake	
	25 g to 30 g of fiber per day.

SPECIAL PROCEDURES

Measure mid–upper arm circumference (MAC)

Place tape around upper right arm, midway between tips of olecranon and acromial processes. Hold tape snugly and make the reading to nearest 5 mm.	**EXPECTED:** Between 10th and 95th percentiles. **UNEXPECTED:** Less than 10th or greater than 95th percentile (see table below).

Percentiles for Midarm Circumference, Midarm Muscle Circumference, and Triceps Skinfold

	Men		Women	
Percentile	55–65 years	65–75 years	55–65 years	65–75 years
Arm Circumference (MAC), cm				
10th	27.3	26.3	25.7	25.2
50th	31.7	30.7	30.3	29.9
95th	36.9	35.5	38.5	37.3
Arm Muscle Circumference (MAMC), cm				
10th	24.5	23.5	19.6	19.5
50th	27.8	26.8	22.5	22.5
95th	32.0	30.6	28.0	27.9
Triceps Skinfold (TSF), mm				
10th	6	6	16	14
50th	11	11	25	24
95th	22	22	38	36

From Frisancho AR, 1981.

TECHNIQUE   **FINDINGS**

This measurement is used along with the tricipeps skinfold thickness to calculate midarm muscle circumference (MAMC).

Measure triceps skinfold (TSF) thickness

Have patient flex right arm at a right angle. Find midpoint between tips of olecranon and acromial process, and make a horizontal mark. Then draw a vertical line to intersect. With arm relaxed, use your thumb and forefinger to grasp and lift triceps skinfold about $1/2$ inch proximal to intersection marks. Place caliper at skinfold and measure without making an indentation. Make two readings to nearest millimeter, and derive an average.

This measurement is used along with the MAC to calculate MAMC.

EXPECTED: Between 10th and 95th percentiles.
UNEXPECTED: Less than 10th or greater than 95th percentile (see table on p. 23).

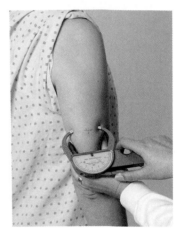

Calculate MAMC

MAMC = {MAC (mm) −
[3.14 × TSF (mm)]}

Compare measurement to table for percentiles.

EXPECTED: Between 10th and 95th percentiles.
UNEXPECTED: Less than 10th or greater than 95th percentile (see table on p. 23).

BIOCHEMICAL MEASUREMENTS

Obtain biochemical measures as indicated

Hemoglobin
Hematocrit
Serum albumin
Transferrin saturation

EXPECTED: See reference ranges established by your particular laboratory.

TECHNIQUE	FINDINGS
Serum glucose	
Triglycerides	
Cholesterol	
High-density lipoprotein (HDL) cholesterol	
Low-density lipoprotein (LDL) cholesterol	
Serum folate	

AIDS TO DIFFERENTIAL DIAGNOSIS

ABNORMALITY	DESCRIPTION
Obesity	Exogenous obesity characterized by excess fat located in breast, buttocks, thighs. Associated with excessive caloric intake, thick skin, pale striae, preservation of muscle strength, no evidence of osteoporosis. Endogenous obesity characterized by excess fat tissue distributed to certain regions of the body such as trunk or abdominal areas.
Anorexia nervosa	Psychologic disorder in which patient has a relentless drive for thinness through self-imposed starvation, bizarre food habits, obsessive exercise, self-induced vomiting or laxative abuse. Condition characterized by weight loss to 85% or less of expected weight or failure to attain expected weight. Common signs and symptoms include those of starvation.
Bulimia	Eating disorder characterized by binge eating, followed by self-induced vomiting. Patient usually does not become malnourished unless body weight continues to drop to less than 85% of expected weight.

TECHNIQUE	FINDINGS
Anemias	Lowering of serum hemoglobin and hematocrit levels and change in size, appearance, and production of red blood cells; common symptoms include pallor, weakness, fatigue, headache, dizziness (see table on p. 27).
Hyperlipidemia	High blood cholesterol (240 g/100 mL) defined as value above which risk for coronary heart disease sharply rises (see box below and table on p. 29).

PEDIATRIC VARIATIONS

EXAMINATION

TECHNIQUE	FINDINGS

MEASURE HEAD CIRCUMFERENCE

Wrap tape measure snugly around infant's head at occipital protuberance and supraorbital prominence.	Refer to growth charts for infants and children.

CALCULATE ESTIMATES FOR ENERGY NEEDS

	Pediatric patients: 1000 kcal plus 100 kcal per year of age, up to age 12 years. *Fat:* Over age 2 years, less than 30% of daily calories from fat; before age 2 years, fat intake of 35% to 40% of calories.

Comparison of Laboratory Test Results for Anemias

Test	Normal Value	Iron Deficiency Anemia	Folic Acid Deficiency Anemia	Vitamin B_{12} Deficiency Anemia
Hemoglobin, 100 g/mL	Men: 14-16 Women: 12-14	Decreased	Decreased	Decreased
Hematocrit, %	Men: 40-54 Women: 37-47	Decreased	Decreased	Decreased
Mean corpuscular volume (MCV), mcg^3	82-92	Decreased (<80)	Increased (>92)	Increased (>92)
Mean corpuscular hemoglobin (MCH), pg	27-31	Decreased (<27)	Increased (>35)	Increased (>35)
Mean corpuscular hemoglobin concentration (MCHC), %	32-36	Decreased (<32)	Normal	Normal
Serum iron, mcg/100 mL	60-180	Decreased	Increased	Increased
Total iron-binding capacity (TIBC), mcg/100 mL	250-450	Increased (>350)	Normal	Normal
Transferrin saturation, %	20-55	Decreased (<20)	Normal	Normal

SAMPLE DOCUMENTATION

Subjective. A 45-year-old business man with steady weight gain over the past 5 years. Seeks nutrition counseling for weight loss plan. Eats three full meals each day with snacking in between; eats breakfast and dinner at home, where wife prepares meals. Often eats lunch (fast foods) on the run. Alcohol intake: 1 to 2 glasses of wine daily with dinner. No regular exercise. Has never kept a meal log. No change in lifestyle; moderate stress.

Objective. Height: 173 cm (68 inches). Weight: 90.9 kg (200 pounds), 123% of desirable body weight; BMI: 30.5; triceps skinfold thickness: 20 mm, 90th percentile; midarm circumference: 327.8 mm; midarm muscle circumference: 26.5 cm, 25th percentile; waist circumference: 42 inches; hip circumference: 41 inches; waist-to-hip ratio: 1.02; 2200 calories daily estimated for appropriate weight loss.

AIDS TO DIFFERENTIAL DIAGNOSIS

Risk Categories and Associated LDL-C Goals from the ATP (Adult Treatment Panel) III Update 2004

Risk Category	Risk Quantification	Factors	LDL-C Goal
High risk	Coronary heart disease (CHD) (10-year risk >20%)* or CHD risk equivalents (10-year risk >20%)	History of myocardial infarction, unstable angina, stable angina, coronary artery procedures (angioplasty or bypass surgery), or evidence of clinically significant myocardial ischemia Clinical manifestations of noncoronary forms of atherosclerotic disease (peripheral arterial disease, abdominal aortic aneurysm, and carotid artery disease [transient ischemic attacks or stroke of carotid origin or >50% obstruction of a carotid artery]), diabetes 2+ risk factors with 10-year risk for hard CHD >20%.[†]	<100 mg/dL (optional goals: <70 mg/dL) <100 mg/dL (optional goals: <70 mg/dL)
Moderately high risk	2+ risk factors (10-year risk 10% to 20%)	Cigarette smoking, hypertension (BP >140/90 mm Hg or on antihypertensive medication), low HDL cholesterol (<40 mg/dL),	<130 mg/dL (optional goal <100 mg/dL)
Moderate risk	2+ risk factors (10-year risk <10%)	family history of premature CHD (CHD in male first-degree relative <55 years of age; CHD in female first-degree relative <65 years of age),	<130 mg/dL
Low risk	0-1 risk factors	age (men >45 years; women >55 years).	<160 mg/dL

From Grundy et al, 2004.
*Electronic 10-year risk calculators are available at www.nhlbi.nih.gov/guidelines/cholesterol
HDL cholesterol ≥60 mg/dL counts as a negative risk factor; its presence removes one risk factor from the total count.
In ATP III, diabetes is regarded as a CHD risk equivalent.
[†]Hard CHD = myocardial infarction and CHD deaths

Clinical Signs and Symptoms of Various Nutrient Deficiencies

Examination	Sign/Symptom	Deficiency
Hair	Alopecia	Zinc, essential fatty acids
	Easy pluckability	Protein, essential fatty acids
	Lackluster	Protein, zinc
	"Corkscrew" hair	Vitamin C, vitamin A
	Decreased pigmentation	Protein, copper
Eyes	Xerosis of conjunctiva	Vitamin A
	Corneal vascularization	Riboflavin
	Keratomalacia	Vitamin A
	Bitot spots	Vitamin A
GI tract	Nausea, vomiting	Pyridoxine
	Diarrhea	Zinc, niacin
	Stomatitis	Pyridoxine, riboflavin, iron
	Cheilosis	Pyridoxine, iron
	Glossitis	Pyridoxine, zinc, niacin, folate, vitamin B_{12}
		Riboflavin
		Vitamin C
		Niacin
		Protein
Skin	Dry and scaling	Vitamin A, essential fatty acids, zinc
	Petechiae/ecchymoses	Vitamin A, vitamin K
	Follicular hyperkeratosis	Vitamin C, vitamin K
	Nasolabial seborrhea	Vitamin A, essential fatty acids
	Bilateral dermatitis	Niacin, pyridoxine, riboflavin Niacin, zinc
Extremities	Subcutaneous fat loss	Kcalories
	Muscle wastage	Kcalories, protein
	Edema	Protein
	Osteomalacia, bone pain, rickets	Vitamin D
	Arthralgia	Vitamin C
Neurologic	Disorientation	Niacin, thiamine
	Confabulation	Thiamine
	Neuropathy	Thiamine, pyridoxine, chromium
	Paresthesia	Thiamine, pyridoxine, vitamin B_{12}
Cardiovascular	Congestive heart failure, cardiomegaly, tachycardia	Thiamine
	Cardiomyopathy	Selenium

Data from Ross Products Division, Abbott Laboratories Inc.

Staying Well

Therapeutic Lifestyle Changes

ATP III recommends a multifaceted lifestyle approach to reduce risk for CHD. This approach is designated *therapeutic lifestyle changes (TLC)*. Its essential features are:

- Reduced intakes of saturated fats (<7% of total calories) and cholesterol (<200 mg per day) (see below for nutrient composition of the TLC Diet)
- Therapeutic options for enhancing LDL lowering such as plant stanols/sterols (2 g/day) and increased viscous (soluble) fiber (10-25 g/day)
- Weight reduction
- Increased physical activity

Nutrient Composition of the TLC Diet

Nutrient	Recommended Intake
Saturated fat*	Less than 7% of total calories
Polyunsaturated fat	Up to 10% of total calories
Monounsaturated fat	Up to 20% of total calories
Total fat	25-35% of total calories
Carbohydrate[†]	50-60% of total calories
Fiber	20-30 g/day
Protein	Approximately 15% of total calories
Cholesterol	Less than 200 mg/day
Total calories (energy)[‡s]	Balance energy intake and expenditure to maintain desirable body weight/prevent weight gain

From ATP III, JAMA 2001.
*Trans fatty acids are another LDL-raising fat that should be kept at a low intake.
†Carbohydrate should be derived predominantly from foods rich in complex carbohydrates including grains, especially whole grains, fruits, and vegetables.
‡Daily energy expenditure should include at least moderate physical activity (contributing approximately 200 kcal per day).

SKIN, HAIR, AND NAILS

EQUIPMENT

- Centimeter ruler (flexible, clear)
- Flashlight with transilluminator
- Wood's lamp (to view fluorescing lesions)
- Handheld magnifying lens (optional)

EXAMINATION

TECHNIQUE   **FINDINGS**

SKIN

Perform overall inspection of entire body

In particular, check areas not usually exposed and intertriginous surfaces.

EXPECTED: Skin color differences among body areas and between sun-exposed and non-sun-exposed areas.
UNEXPECTED: Lesions.

Inspect skin of each body area and mucous membranes

- *Color/uniformity*
  Inspect sclerae, conjunctivae, buccal mucosa, tongue, lips, nail beds, and palms of dark-skinned patients for color hues.

EXPECTED: General uniformity—dark brown to light tan, with pink or yellow overtones. Sun-darkened areas. Darker skin around knees and elbows. Calloused areas yellow. Knuckles darker and palms/soles lighter in dark-skinned patients. Vascular flush areas pink or red, especially with anxiety or excitement.

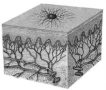

Spider angioma—red central body with radiating spiderlike legs that blanch with pressure to the central body
Cause: Liver disease, vitamin B deficiency, idiopathic

Purpura—red-purple nonblanchable discoloration greater than 0.5 cm diameter.
Cause: Intravascular defects, infection

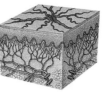

Venous star—bluish spider, linear or irregularly shaped; does not blanch with pressure
Cause: Increased pressure in superficial veins

Petechiae—red-purple nonblanchable discoloration less than 0.5 cm diameter
Cause: Intravascular defects, infection

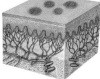

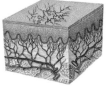

Telangiectasia—fine, irregular red line
Cause: Dilation of capillaries

Ecchymoses—red-purple nonblanchable discoloration of variable size
Cause: Vascular wall destruction, trauma, vasculitis

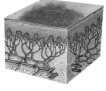

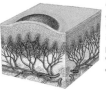

Capillary hemangioma (nevus flammeus)—red irregular macular patches
Cause: Dilation of dermal capillaries

Cutaneous Color Changes

Color	Cause	Distribution	Select Conditions
Brown	Darkening of melanin pigment	Generalized	Pituitary, adrenal, liver disease Nevi, neurofibromatosis
White	Absence of	Generalized Localized	Albinism Vitiligo
Red (erythema)	Increased cutaneous blood flow	Localized Generalized	Inflammation Fever, viral exanthems, urticaria
	Increased intravascular red blood cells	Generalized	Polycythemia

Continued

Cutaneous Color Changes—cont'd

Color	Cause	Distribution	Select Conditions
Yellow	Increased bile pigmentation (jaundice)	Generalized	Liver disease
	Increased carotene pigmentation	Generalized (except sclera)	Hypothyroidism, increased intake of vegetables containing carotene
	Decreased visibility of oxyhemoglobin	Generalized	Anemia, chronic renal disease
Blue	Increased unsaturated hemoglobin secondary to hypoxia	Lips, mouth, nail beds	Cardiovascular and pulmonary disease

TECHNIQUE	**FINDINGS**
	Pigmented nevi. Nonpigmented striae. Freckles. Birthmarks. **UNEXPECTED:** Dysplastic, precancerous, or cancerous nevi. Chloasma. Unpigmented skin. Generalized or localized color changes. Vascular skin lesions. Vascular changes.
■ *Thickness*	**EXPECTED:** Thickness variations, with eyelids thinnest, areas of rubbing thickest. Calluses on hands and feet. **UNEXPECTED:** Atrophy. Hyperkeratosis.
■ *Symmetry*	**EXPECTED:** Bilateral symmetry.
■ *Hygiene*	**EXPECTED:** Clean.
Palpate skin	
■ *Moisture*	**EXPECTED:** Minimal perspiration or oiliness. Increased perspiration (associated with activity, environment, obesity, anxiety, excitement) noticeable on palms, scalp, forehead, axillae.

TECHNIQUE	**FINDINGS**
	UNEXPECTED: Damp intertriginous areas.
▣ *Temperature* Palpate with dorsal surface of hand or fingers.	**EXPECTED:** Cool to warm. Bilateral symmetry.
▣ *Texture*	**EXPECTED:** Smooth, soft, and even. Roughness resulting from heavy clothing, cold weather, or soap. **UNEXPECTED:** Extensive or widespread roughness.
▣ *Turgor and mobility* Gently pinch skin on forearm or in sternal area and release.	**EXPECTED:** Resilience. **UNEXPECTED:** Failure of skin to return to place quickly.

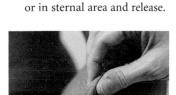

Inspect and palpate lesions

▣ *Size*
Measure all dimensions.   **UNEXPECTED:** See table on pp. 36–39.

Text continues on p. 40.

Primary Skin Lesions

Description	Examples

Macule

Flat, circumscribed area that is a change in skin color; less than 1 cm in diameter

Freckles, flat moles (nevi), petechiae, measles, scarlet fever

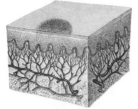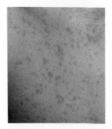

Measles. *From Habif, 2004.*

Papule

Elevated, firm, circumscribed area less than 1 cm in diameter

Wart (verruca), elevated moles, lichen planus

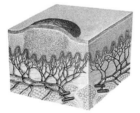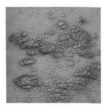

Lichen planus. *From Weston, Lane, Morelli, 1996.*

Patch

Flat, nonpalpable, irregular-shaped macule more than 1 cm in diameter

Vitiligo, port-wine stains, mongolian spots, café au lait spots

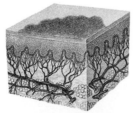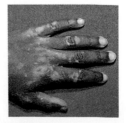

Vitiligo. *From Weston, Lane, and Morelli, 1991.*

Primary Skin Lesions—cont'd

Description	Examples

Plaque

Elevated, firm, and rough lesion with flat top surface greater than I cm in diameter

Psoriasis, seborrheic and actinic keratoses

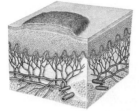

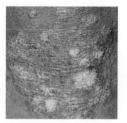

Plaque. *From Habif, 2004.*

Wheal

Elevated irregular-shaped area of cutaneous edema; solid, transient; variable diameter

Insect bites, urticaria, allergic reaction

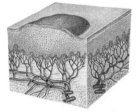

Wheal. *From Farrar et al, 1992.*

Nodule

Elevated, firm, circumscribed lesion; deeper in dermis than a papule; I to 2 cm in diameter

Erythema nodosum, lipomas

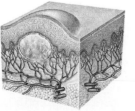

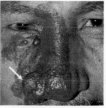

Hypertrophic nodule. *From Goldman and Fitzpatrick, 1999.*

Continued

Primary Skin Lesions—cont'd

Description	Examples

Tumor

Elevated and solid lesion; may or may not be clearly demarcated; deeper in dermis; greater than 2 cm in diameter

Neoplasms, benign tumor, lipoma, hemangioma

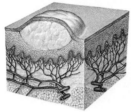 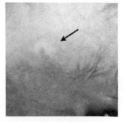

Hemangioma. *From Weston, Lane, Morelli, 1996.*

Vesicle

Elevated, circumscribed, superficial, not into dermis; filled with serous fluid; less than 1 cm in diameter

Varicella (chickenpox), herpes zoster (shingles)

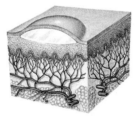 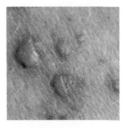

Vesicles caused by varicella. *From Farrar et al, 1992.*

Bulla

Vesicle greater than 1 cm in diameter

Blister, pemphigus vulgaris

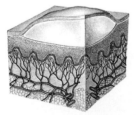 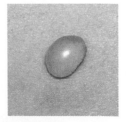

Blister. *From White, 1994.*

Primary Skin Lesions—cont'd

Description	Examples

Pustule

Elevated, superficial lesion; similar to a vesicle but filled with purulent fluid

Impetigo, acne

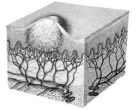

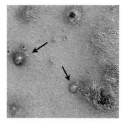

Acne. *From Weston, Lane, Morelli, 1996.*

Cyst

Elevated, circumscribed, encapsulated lesion; in dermis or subcutaneous layer; filled with liquid or semisolid material

Sebaceous cyst, cystic acne

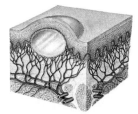

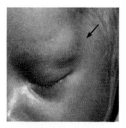

Sebaceous cyst. *From Weston, Lane, Morelli, 1996.*

Telangiectasia

Fine, irregular red lines produced by capillary dilation

Telangiectasia in rosacea

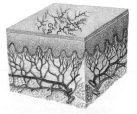

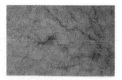

Telangiectasia. *From Lemmi, Lemmi, 2000.*

TECHNIQUE	FINDINGS

Inspect and palpate lesions—cont'd

- *Shape*
- *Color*
  Use Wood's lamp to distinguish fluorescing lesions.
- *Blanching*
- *Texture*
  Transilluminate to determine presence of fluid.
- *Elevation/depression*
- *Pedunculation*
- *Exudate*
  Note color, odor, amount, and consistency of lesion.
- *Configuration*
  Check lesion for annular, grouped, linear, arciform, or diffuse arrangement.
- *Location/distribution*
  Check lesion for generalized/localized, body region, patterns, or discrete/confluent.

HAIR

Inspect hair over entire body

- *Color*

  EXPECTED: Light blond to black and gray, with alterations caused by rinses, dyes, and permanents.

- *Distribution/quantity*

  EXPECTED: Hair present on scalp, lower face, neck, nares, ears, chest, axillae, back and shoulders, arms, legs, pubic areas, and around nipples. Scalp hair loss in adult men, adrenal androgenic female-pattern alopecia in adult women.

  UNEXPECTED: Localized or generalized hair loss, inflammation, or scarring. Broken/absent hair shafts. Hirsutism in women.

TECHNIQUE	**FINDINGS**

Palpate for texture

EXPECTED: Coarse or fine, curly or straight, shiny, smooth, and resilient. Fine vellus covering body; coarse terminal hair on scalp, on pubis, on axillary areas, and in male beard.
UNEXPECTED: Dryness and brittleness.

NAILS

Inspect nails

■ *Color*

EXPECTED: Variations of pink with varying opacity. Pigment deposits in persons with dark skin. White spots.
UNEXPECTED: Yellow or green-black discoloration. Diffuse darkening. Pigment deposits in persons with light skin. Longitudinal red, brown, or white streaks or white bands. White, yellow, or green tinge. Blue nail beds. Blue-black discoloration.

■ *Length/configuration/ symmetry*

EXPECTED: Varying shape, smooth and flat/slightly convex, with edges smooth and rounded.
UNEXPECTED: Jagged, broken, or bitten edges or cuticles. Peeling. Absence of nail.

■ *Cleanliness*

EXPECTED: Clean and neat.
UNEXPECTED: Unkempt

■ *Ridging and beading*

EXPECTED: Longitudinal ridging and beading.
UNEXPECTED: Longitudinal ridging and grooving with lichen planus. Transverse grooving, rippling, and depressions. Pitting.

TECHNIQUE   **FINDINGS**

Palpate nail plate

- *Texture/firmness/thickness/ uniformity*

EXPECTED: Hard and smooth with uniform thickness.
UNEXPECTED: Thickening or thinning.

- *Adherence to nail bed* Gently squeeze between thumb and finger.

EXPECTED: Firmness.
UNEXPECTED: Separation. Boggy nail base.

Measure nail base angle

Inspect fingers when patient places dorsal surfaces of fingertips together.

EXPECTED: 160-degree angle.
UNEXPECTED: Clubbing.

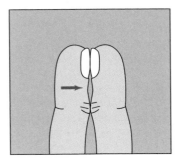

Expected finding

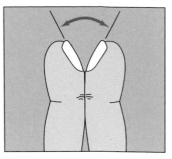

Clubbing

Inspect and palpate proximal and lateral nail folds

UNEXPECTED: Redness, swelling, pus, warts, cysts, tumors, and pain.

AIDS TO DIFFERENTIAL DIAGNOSIS

ABNORMALITY	DESCRIPTION
Corn (clavus)	Flat or slightly elevated, circumscribed, painful lesions. Smooth, hard surface. Soft corns—whitish thickenings. Hard corns—sharply delineated, conical.

ABNORMALITY	DESCRIPTION
Callus	Superficial area of hyperkeratosis. Less demarcated than corns. Usually nontender.
Tinea (dermatophytosis)	Papular, pustular, vesicular, erythematous, or scaling lesions. Possible secondary bacterial infection.
Basal cell carcinoma	Cutaneous neoplasm in nodular, pigmented, cystic, sclerosing, superficial, and other forms.
Squamous cell carcinoma	Cutaneous neoplasm that appears soft, mobile, and elevated with a surface scale. The base of the lesion may be inflamed.
Malignant melanoma	Cutaneous neoplasm that presents with characteristic asymmetry, irregular borders, variegated colors, and is growing or larger than 6 mm (see ABCDs of Melanoma on p. 48).
Kaposi sarcoma	Soft, vascular, blue-purple, painless lesions. Macular or papular. May appear as plaques, keloids, or ecchymotic areas.
Eczematous dermatitis	Acute—erythematous, pruritic, weeping vesicles, often excoriated and crusted from scratching. Subacute—erythema and scaling, possible itching. Chronic—thick, lichenified, pruritic plaques.
Paronychia	Redness, swelling, tenderness at lateral and proximal nail folds. Possible purulent drainage under cuticle. Acute or chronic (with nail rippling).
Ingrown nail	Pain and swelling resulting from nail piercing fold and growing into dermis.

AIDS TO DIFFERENTIAL DIAGNOSIS

Cutaneous Manifestations of Two Pathogens That May Be Used in Biologic Warfare

Disease	Pathogen	Communicability	Incubation	Skin Lesions	Accompanying Symptoms
Cutaneous anthrax*	Spore-forming bacterium *Bacillus anthracis*	Direct person-to-person spread extremely unlikely	Up to 12 days following deposition of organism into skin with previous abrasion	Pruritic macule or papule that enlarges into a round ulcer by day 2. Central necrosis develops with a painless ulcer covered by black eschar, which dries and falls off in 1-2 weeks. May be accompanied by 1 to 3 mm vesicles that discharge clear or serosanguineous fluid	Lymphangitis; lymphadenopathy

A gram-stained smear of material taken from the lesion will reveal the gram-positive rods of *Bacillus anthracis*. *From Beeching, Nye, 1996.*

Respiratory and gastrointestinal forms of anthrax also exist.

Cutaneous Manifestations of Two Pathogens That May Be Used in Biologic Warfare—cont'd

Disease	Pathogen	Communicability	Incubation	Skin Lesions	Accompanying Symptoms
Smallpox	Variola virus	Direct transmission by infected saliva droplets. Most infectious during the first week of illness. However, some risk of transmission lasts until all scabs have fallen off. Contaminated clothing or bed linen could also spread the virus.	12 days (range: 7-17 days) following exposure	Rash appears 2-3 days after systemic symptoms, first on the mucosa of the mouth and pharynx, face, and forearms, spreading to the trunk and legs. Starts with flat red lesions that evolve at the same rate (compared with varicella, which matures in crops). Lesions become vesicular, then pustular and begin to crust early in the second week.	Initial systemic symptoms include high fever, fatigue, headache, and backache.

Smallpox. This archival photograph shows eczema vaccinatum acquired from a relative who had recently been vaccinated against smallpox.

From Beeching, Nye, 1996.

PEDIATRIC VARIATIONS

EXAMINATION

TECHNIQUE	FINDINGS

SKIN

Inspect hands and feet of newborns for skin creases

EXPECTED: Number of creases is indication of maturity of newborn; the older the gestational age, the more creases.
UNEXPECTED: Single transverse crease across palm frequently seen in infants with Down syndrome.

AIDS TO DIFFERENTIAL DIAGNOSIS

ABNORMALITY	DESCRIPTION
Café au lait spots	Coffee-colored multiple patches, diameter more than 1 cm.
Seborrheic dermatitis	Thick, yellow, adherent crusted scalp, ear, or neck lesions.
Impetigo	Honey-colored crusted or ruptured vesicles.
Miliaria ("prickly heat")	Irregular, red, macular rash.
Reddened patches	Irregular reddened areas suggestive of richer capillary bed. Include strawberry hemangioma and cavernous hemangioma.
Chickenpox (varicella)	Fever, mild malaise, and pruritic maculopapular skin eruption that becomes vesicular in a matter of hours.
German measles (rubella)	Generalized light pink to red maculopapular rash, low-grade fever, coryza, sore throat, cough.

SAMPLE DOCUMENTATION

Subjective. An 18-year-old female with a body rash. First noticed the rash 4 days ago. Thinks it may be from drinking new citrus juice. Describes rash as red and itchy, with transient bumps on face, neck, arms, legs, torso. No known food allergies. Denied exposure to new contact irritants. No new medications; is currently taking antihistamine for allergic rhinitis. Denies respiratory difficulty, difficulty swallowing, edema. Denies fever, cough, malaise.

Objective. *Skin:* Dark pink maculopapular lesions on face, torso, extremities; large urticarial wheal on right cheek. No excoriation or secondary infection. Turgor resilient. Skin uniformly warm and dry. No edema.

Hair: Curly, black, thick with female distribution pattern. Texture coarse.

Nails: Opaque, short, well-groomed, uniform and without deformities. Nail bed pink. Nail base angle 160 degrees. No redness, exudates, or swelling in surrounding folds and no tenderness to palpation.

The ABCDs of Melanoma

Characteristics that should alert you to the possibility of malignant melanoma:

A Asymmetry of lesion. One-half of a mole or birthmark does not match the other.

B Borders. Edges are irregular ragged, notched, or blurred. Pigment may be streaming from the border.

C Color. The color is not the same all over and may have differing shades of brown or black, sometimes with patches of red, white, or blue.

D Diameter. The diameter is larger than 6 mm (about the size of a pencil eraser) or is growing larger.

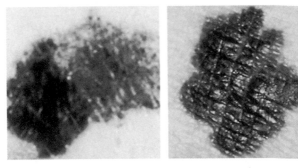

Asymmetry   Border

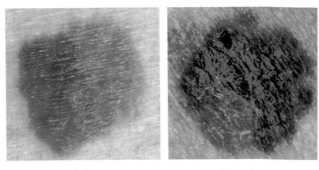

Color   Diameter

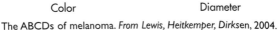

The ABCDs of melanoma. *From Lewis, Heitkemper, Dirksen, 2004.*

LYMPHATIC SYSTEM

EQUIPMENT

- Centimeter ruler
- Skin-marking pencil

EXAMINATION

Lymphatic system is examined by inspection and palpation, region by region, during the examination of other body systems, as well as with palpation of the spleen.

Lymph Nodes Most Accessible to Inspection and Palpation

The more superficial the node, the more accessible it is to your palpation.

"Necklace" of Nodes
Parotid and retropharyngeal (tonsillar)
Submandibular
Submental
Sublingual (facial)
Superficial anterior cervical
Superficial posterior cervical
Preauricular and postauricular
Occipital
Supraclavicular

Arms
Axillary
Epitrochlear (cubital)

Legs
Superficial superior inguinal
Superficial inferior inguinal
Occasionally, popliteal

TECHNIQUE	FINDINGS

HEAD AND NECK

Inspect visible nodes
Ask if patient is aware of any
lumps.

UNEXPECTED: Edema,
erythema, red streaks, or
lesions.

**Palpate superficial nodes; note size, consistency, mobility,
tenderness, warmth**

Bend patient's head slightly
forward or to side. Palpate gently
with pads of second, third,
fourth fingers.

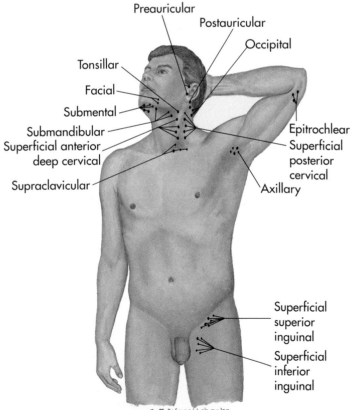

Preauricular
Postauricular
Occipital
Tonsillar
Facial
Submental
Submandibular
Superficial anterior
deep cervical
Supraclavicular
Epitrochlear
Superficial
posterior
cervical
Axillary
Superficial
superior
inguinal
Superficial
inferior
inguinal

G. J. Wassilchenko

TECHNIQUE   **FINDINGS**

HEAD/NECK

- *Occipital nodes at base of skull*
- *Postauricular nodes over mastoid process*
- *Preauricular nodes in front of ears*
- *Parotid and retropharyngeal nodes at angle of mandible*

- *Submandibular nodes between angle and tip of mandible*
- *Submental nodes behind tip of mandible*

EXPECTED: Nodes accessible to palpation but not large or firm enough to be felt.
UNEXPECTED: Enlarged, tender, red or discolored, fixed, matted, inflamed, or warm nodes, increased vascularity.

Preauricular
Parotid
Retropharyngeal (tonsillar)
Submandibular
Submental
Occipital
Postauricular
Posterior cervical
Anterior cervical
Supraclavicular nodes (palpable when there is disease)

NECK

- *Superficial cervical nodes at sternocleidomastoid*
- *Posterior cervical nodes along anterior border of trapezius*
- *Deep cervical nodes along anterior border of trapezius*

EXPECTED: Nodes accessible to palpation but not large or firm enough to be felt.
UNEXPECTED: Enlarged, tender, red or discolored, fixed, matted, inflamed, or warm nodes, increased vascularity.

TECHNIQUE	FINDINGS

UNEXPECTED: Detection of Virchow nodes.

■ *Supraclavicular areas*
If enlarged nodes are found, inspect regions drained by nodes for infection or malignancy and examine other regions for enlargement.

NOTE: A palpable supraclavicular node should always make you suspect the probability of a malignancy.

AXILLAE

Inspect visible nodes

Ask if patient is aware of any lumps.

UNEXPECTED: Edema, erythema, red streaks, or lesions.

Palpate superficial nodes for size, consistency, mobility, tenderness, warmth

Using firm, deliberate, gentle touch, rotate fingertips and palm. Attempt to glide fingers beneath nodes.

Axillary nodes

Support patient's forearm with your contralateral arm, and bring palm of examining hand flat into axilla.

If enlarged nodes are found, inspect regions drained by nodes for infection or malignancy, and examine other regions for enlargement.

EXPECTED: Nodes accessible to palpation but not large or firm enough to be felt.
UNEXPECTED: Enlarged, tender, red or discolored, fixed, matted, inflamed, or warm nodes, increased vascularity.

TECHNIQUE   **FINDINGS**

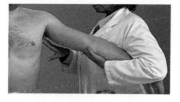

OTHER LYMPH NODES

Inspect visible nodes

Ask if patient is aware of any
lumps.

UNEXPECTED: Edema,
erythema, red streaks, or lesions.

Palpate superficial nodes for size, consistency, mobility, tenderness, warmth

Systematically palpate other areas,
moving hand in circular fashion,
probing without pressing hard.

EXPECTED: Nodes accessible
to palpation but not large or
firm enough to be felt.
UNEXPECTED: Enlarged,
tender, red or discolored, fixed,
matted, inflamed, or warm
nodes, increased vascularity.

■ *Epitrochlear nodes*
  Support elbow in one hand
  while exploring with other.

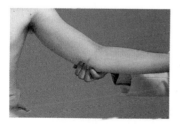

■ *Inguinal and popliteal area*
  Have patient lie supine with
  knee slightly flexed.

TECHNIQUE   FINDINGS

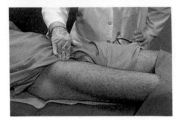

If enlarged nodes are found,
inspect regions drained by nodes
for infection or malignancy and
examine other regions for
enlargement.

AIDS TO DIFFERENTIAL DIAGNOSIS	
ABNORMALITY	**DESCRIPTION**
Acute lymphangitis	Pain, malaise, illness, possibly fever. Red streak (tracing of fine lines) may follow course of lymphatic collecting duct. Inflamed area sometimes slightly indurated and palpable to gentle touch. Related infection possible distally, particularly interdigitally.
Non-Hodgkin lymphoma	Well-defined, solid neoplasm, often in lymph nodes or spleen.
Hodgkin disease	Painless, inexorably progressive enlargement of cervical lymph nodes. Generally asymmetric. Nodes sometimes matted and generally very firm, almost rubbery. Nodes sometimes produce pressure on surrounding structures, prompting need for medical care.
Epstein-Barr virus; mononucleosis	Pharyngitis, fever, fatigue, malaise. Frequently splenomegaly and/or rash.

TECHNIQUE	FINDINGS
	Palpable nodes generalized but more commonly in anterior and posterior cervical chains. Nodes vary in firmness, are generally discrete, are occasionally tender.
Streptococcal pharyngitis	Sore throat. Often runny nose. Sometimes headache, fatigue, abdominal pain. Firm, discrete, often tender anterior cervical nodes generally felt.
Herpes simplex	Often discrete labial and gingival ulcers, high fever, enlargement of anterior cervical and submandibular nodes. Nodes tend to be firm, quite discrete, movable, tender.
Acquired immunodeficiency syndrome (AIDS)	Recurrent, often severe, opportunistic infections. Initially lymphadenopathy, fatigue, fever, weight loss.
Human immunodeficiency virus (HIV) seropositivity	Warning signs: severe fatigue, malaise, weakness, persistent unexplained weight loss, persistent lymphadenopathy, fevers, arthralgias, persistent diarrhea.

Some Conditions Simulating Lymph Node Enlargement

Lymphangioma
Hemangioma (tends to feel spongy; appears reddish blue, depending on size and extent of angiomatous involvement)
Branchial cleft cyst (sometimes accompanied by tiny orifice in neck on line extending to ear)

Thyroglossal duct cyst
Laryngocele
Esophageal diverticulum
Thyroid goiter
Graves disease
Hashimoto thyroiditis
Parotid swelling (e.g., from mumps or tumor)

PEDIATRIC VARIATIONS

EXAMINATION

TECHNIQUE   **FINDINGS**

HEAD AND NECK

Palpate superficial nodes

■ *Occipital nodes at base of skull*

■ *Postauricular nodes over mastoid process*

EXPECTED: In children, small, firm, discrete, nontender, nonmovable nodes in occipital, postauricular chains.

OTHER LYMPH NODES

Palpate superficial nodes

■ *Inguinal and popliteal area*

EXPECTED: In children, small, firm, discrete nodes; nontender, movable in inguinal chain.

SAMPLE DOCUMENTATION

Subjective. A 25-year-old woman complains of difficulty swallowing and sore throat for 3 days, now subsiding. Fever to 38° C (100.5° F) for 2 days. Has been using acetaminophen and throat lozenges for pain relief.

Objective. No visible enlargement of lymph nodes in any area. Enlarged node (2 cm in diameter) palpated in left posterior cervical triangle; firm, nontender, movable, no overlying warmth, erythema, or edema. A few shotty nodes palpated in posterior cervical triangles bilaterally and in femoral chains bilaterally.

EQUIPMENT

- Tape measure
- Cup of water
- Stethoscope
- Transilluminator

EXAMINATION

Ask patient to sit.

TECHNIQUE   **FINDINGS**

HEAD AND FACE

Observe head position

EXPECTED: Upright, midline, still.
UNEXPECTED: Horizontal jerking or bobbing, nodding, tilted.

Inspect facial features

- *Shape*
  Observe eyelids, eyebrows, palpebral fissures, nasolabial folds, mouth at rest, during movement, with expression.

EXPECTED: Variations according to race, sex, age, body build.
UNEXPECTED: Change in shape. Unusual features: edema, puffiness, coarsened features, prominent eyes, hirsutism, lack of expression, excessive

TECHNIQUE	FINDINGS
	perspiration, pallor, or pigmentation variations. Tics.
■ *Symmetry* Note if asymmetry affects all features of one side or a portion of face.	**EXPECTED:** Slight asymmetry. **UNEXPECTED:** Facial nerve paralysis, facial nerve weakness, or problem with peripheral trigeminal nerve.
■ *Characteristic facies*	

Inspect skull and scalp

■ *Size/shape/symmetry* ■ *Scalp condition* ■ *Systematically part hair from frontal to occipital region.* ■ *Hair pattern* Pay special attention to areas behind ears, at hairline, at crown.	**EXPECTED:** Symmetric. **UNEXPECTED:** Lesions, scabs, tenderness, parasites, nits, scaliness. **EXPECTED:** Bitemporal recession or balding over crown in men. **UNEXPECTED:** Random areas of alopecia or alopecia totalis.

Palpate head and scalp

■ *Symmetry* Palpate in gentle, rotary motion from front to back.	**EXPECTED:** Symmetric and smooth with bones indistinguishable. Ridge of sagittal fissure occasionally palpable. **UNEXPECTED:** Indentations or depressions.

Palpate hair

■ *Texture/color distribution*	**EXPECTED:** Smooth, symmetrically distributed. **UNEXPECTED:** Splitting or cracked ends. Coarse, dry, or brittle. Fine and silky.

TECHNIQUE	**FINDINGS**

Palpate temporal arteries

Note course of arteries.

UNEXPECTED: Thickening, hardness, or tenderness.

Auscultate temporal arteries and over skull and eyes

EXPECTED: No bruits.

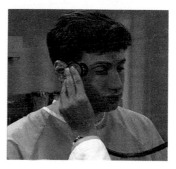

Inspect salivary glands

- *Symmetry/size*
  Palpate if asymmetry noted.
  Have patient open mouth
  and press on salivary duct
  to attempt to express material.

UNEXPECTED: Asymmetry
or enlargement. Tenderness.
Discrete nodule.

NECK

Inspect neck

- *Symmetry*
  Inspect in usual position, in
  slight hyperextension, and
  during swallowing. Look for
  landmarks of anterior and
  posterior triangles.
- *Trachea*
  Inspect in usual position, in
  slight hyperextension,
  and while patient swallows.
- *Condition of neck*

EXPECTED: Bilateral
symmetry of
sternocleidomastoid and
trapezius muscles.
UNEXPECTED: Asymmetry,
torticollis.
EXPECTED: Midline
placement.
UNEXPECTED: Masses,
webbing, excessive posterior
skinfolds, unusually short neck,
distention of jugular vein,
prominence of carotid arteries,
or edema.

TECHNIQUE	FINDINGS

Evaluate range of motion

Have patient flex, extend, rotate, laterally turn head and neck.

EXPECTED: Smooth.
UNEXPECTED: Pain, dizziness, or limitation of motion.

Palpate neck

▪ *Trachea*
Place thumb on each side of trachea in lower portion of neck, and compare space between trachea and sternocleidomastoid on each side.

EXPECTED: Midline position.
UNEXPECTED: Deviation to right or left.

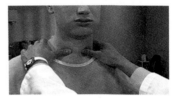

▪ *Hyoid bone/thyroid and cricoid cartilages*
Have patient swallow.
▪ *Cartilaginous rings of trachea*
Have patient swallow.
▪ *Tracheal tug*
With neck extended, palpate for movement with index finger and thumb on each side of trachea below thyroid isthmus.

EXPECTED: Smooth. Moves during swallowing.
UNEXPECTED: Tender.
EXPECTED: Distinct.
UNEXPECTED: Tender.
UNEXPECTED: Tug synchronous with pulse.

Palpate lymph nodes

▪ *Size/consistency, mobility/ condition*

UNEXPECTED: Enlarged, matted, tender, fixed, warm.

Palpate thyroid gland

▪ *Symmetry*
Observe from frontal and lateral positions while patient hyperextends neck. Then

UNEXPECTED: Asymmetry. Enlarged and visible thyroid gland.

TECHNIQUE	**FINDINGS**

observe as patient sips water while neck is hyperextended.

■ *Size/shape/configuration/ consistency*
Stand either facing or behind patient. Have patient hold head slightly forward and tipped toward side being examined. Lightly palpate isthmus and lateral lobes. Give water to patient to facilitate swallowing.
From the front, examine the left lobe by sitting on the left side of the patient and pressing the trachea to the left with the left thumb. Place the first three fingers in the thyroid bed just medial to the sternocleidomastoid. Keep your fingers still while the patient again swallows, thereby moving the gland beneath your fingers.
Repeat on the right side.
    If gland is enlarged, auscultate for vascular sounds with stethoscope bell.

EXPECTED: Lobes (if felt) small and smooth. Gland rises freely with swallowing. Right lobe as much as 25% larger than left. Tissue firm and pliable.
UNEXPECTED: Enlarged, tender nodules (smooth or irregular, soft or hard); coarse tissue; gritty sensation.
UNEXPECTED: Bruit.

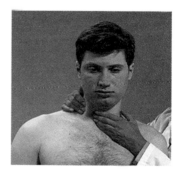

AIDS TO DIFFERENTIAL DIAGNOSIS

ABNORMALITY	DESCRIPTION
Myxedema	Dull, puffy, yellow skin. Coarse, sparse hair. Temporal loss of eyebrows. Periorbital edema. Prominent tongue. Hypothyroidism (see table on p. 63).
Graves disease	Diffuse thyroid enlargement, hyperthyroidism. Various pathologic conditions— ophthalmologic (prominent eyes, lid retraction, staring or startled expression), dermatologic (fine and moist skin, fine hair), musculoskeletal (muscle weakness), cardiac (tachycardia) (see table on p. 63).
Down syndrome	Depressed nasal bridge, epicanthal folds, mongoloid slant of eyes, low-set ears, large tongue.

Hyperthyroidism Versus Hypothyroidism

System or Structure Affected	Hyperthyroidism	Hypothyroidism
Constitutional		
Temperature preference	Cool climate	Warm climate
Weight	Loss	Gain
Emotional state	Nervous, easily irritated, highly energetic	Lethargic, complacent, uninterested
Hair	Fine, with hair loss; failure to hold permanent wave	Coarse, with tendency to break
Skin	Warm, fine, hyperpigmentation at pressure points	Coarse, scaling, dry
Fingernails	Thin, with tendency to break; may show onycholysis	Thick
Eyes	Bilateral or unilateral proptosis, lid retraction, double vision	Puffiness in periorbital region
Neck	Goiter, change in shirt neck size, pain over thyroid	No goiter
Cardiac	Tachycardia, dysrhythmia, palpitations	No change noted
Gastrointestinal	Increased frequency of bowel movements; diarrhea rare	Constipation
Menstrual	Scant flow, amenorrhea	Menorrhagia
Neuromuscular	Increasing weakness, especially of proximal muscles	Lethargic, but good muscular strength

Headaches

Headaches are one of the most common complaints and probably one of the most self-medicated. They are not always benign. A history of insistent headache that is severe and recurrent must always be given attention. Sometimes the underlying cause is life-threatening, such as a brain tumor. Sometimes it is life-intimidating, such as migraines. At other times it is easily confronted, such as when it is the result of drinking wine. The patient's history is fully as important as the physical examination in getting at the root of a headache. Various kinds of headaches can be compared as follows.

Characteristic	Classic Migraine	Common Migraine	Cluster	Hypertensive	Muscular, Tension
Age at onset	Childhood	Childhood	Adulthood	Adulthood	Adulthood
Location	Unilateral	Generalized	Unilateral	Bilateral or occipital	Unilateral or bilateral
Duration	Hours to days	Hours to days	½ to 2 hours	Hours	Hours to days
Time of onset	Morning or night	Morning or night	Night	Morning	Anytime, commonly in afternoon or evening
Quality of pain	Pulsating or throbbing	Pulsating or throbbing	Intense burning, boring, searing, knifelike	Throbbing	Bandlike, constricting
Prodromal event	Well-defined neurologic event, scotoma, aphasia, hemianopsia, aura	Vague neurologic, changes, personality change, fluid retention, appetite loss	Personality changes, sleep disturbances	None	None

Headaches—cont'd

Characteristic	Classic Migraine	Common Migraine	Cluster	Hypertensive	Muscular, Tension
Precipitating event	Menstrual period, missing meals, birth control pills, letdown after stress	Menstrual period, missing meals, birth control pills, letdown after stress	Alcohol consumption	None	Stress, anger, bruxism
Frequency	Twice a week	Twice a week	Several times nightly or several nights, then none	Daily	Daily
Gender predilection	Female	Female	Male	Equal	Equal
Other symptoms	Nausea, vomiting	Nausea, vomiting	Increased lacrimation, nasal discharge	Generally remits as day progresses	None

PEDIATRIC VARIATIONS

EXAMINATION

TECHNIQUE	FINDINGS

HEAD AND FACE

Palpate head and scalp

■ *Symmetry*
  In infants, transilluminate
  skull

EXPECTED: An infant's head circumference is 2 cm greater than chest circumference up to the age of 2 years.
EXPECTED: 2-cm ring of light.

■ *Skull condition*

EXPECTED: In infants, posterior fontanel closed at 2 months; anterior fontanel closed at 18 to 24 months.
UNEXPECTED: Tenderness or depressions; sunken areas; swelling, bulging, or depressed fontanels.

■ *Scalp*

EXPECTED: Free movement.
UNEXPECTED: Fixation of scalp, bulging either on one side or crossing midline of scalp.

Percuss skull

EXPECTED: Macewen sign, cracked-pot sound, is physiologic when fontanels are open.
UNEXPECTED: Macewen sign may indicate increased intracranial pressure after fontanel closure.

TECHNIQUE	FINDINGS

Auscultate temporal arteries and over skull and eyes

EXPECTED: Bruits are common in children up to age 5 years.

NECK

Palpate thyroid gland

■ *Symmetry*

EXPECTED: In children, thyroid gland may be palpable.
UNEXPECTED: Tenderness.

SAMPLE DOCUMENTATION

Head. Held erect and midline. Skull normocephalic, symmetric, smooth without deformities. Facial features symmetric. Salivary glands not inflamed or tender. Temporal artery pulsations visible bilaterally, soft and nontender to palpation. No bruits.

Neck. Trachea midline. No jugular venous distention (JVD) or carotid artery prominence. Thyroid palpable, firm, smooth, not enlarged. Thyroid and cartilages move with swallowing. No nodules or tenderness. No bruits. Full range of motion (ROM) of neck without discomfort.

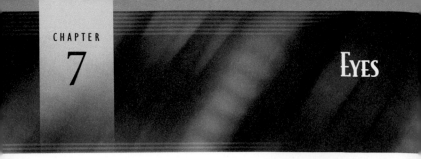

EQUIPMENT

- Snellen chart or Lea cards, Landolt C or HOTV chart
- Eye cover, gauze, or opaque card
- Rosenbaum or Jaeger near-vision card
- Penlight
- Cotton wisp
- Ophthalmoscope

EXAMINATION

Ask patient to sit or stand.

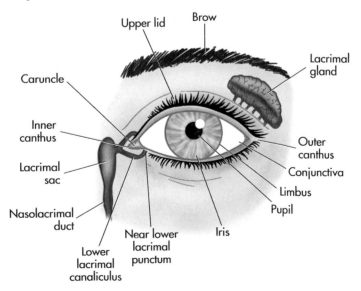

Brow

Upper lid

Lacrimal gland

Caruncle

Inner canthus

Lacrimal sac

Nasolacrimal duct

Outer canthus

Conjunctiva

Limbus

Pupil

Iris

Near lower lacrimal punctum

Lower lacrimal canaliculus

TECHNIQUE   **FINDINGS**

VISUAL TESTING

Measure visual acuity in each eye separately

■ *Distance vision*
Use Snellen chart, Landolt C
or HOTV chart. If testing with
and without corrective lenses,
test without lenses first and
record readings separately.

EXPECTED: Vision 20/20
with or without lenses with near
and far vision in each eye.
UNEXPECTED: Myopia,
amblyopia, or presbyopia.

■ *Near vision*
Use near-vision card.

EXPECTED: Vision 20/20.
UNEXPECTED: Fields of
vision more limited than
temporally, 50 degrees
superiorly, 70 degrees inferiorly.

■ *Peripheral vision*
Test nasal, temporal, superior,
inferior fields by moving your
finger into field from outside.

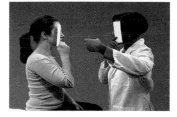

EXTERNAL EXAMINATION

Inspect eyebrows

■ *Size/extension*

EXPECTED: Unusually thin if
plucked.
UNEXPECTED: End short of
temporal canthus.

■ *Hair texture*

UNEXPECTED: Coarse.

Inspect orbital area

UNEXPECTED: Edema,
puffiness not related to aging, or
sagging tissue below orbit.
Xanthelasma.

Inspect eyelids

■ Eyelid position

UNEXPECTED: Ectropion or
entropion.

TECHNIQUE	FINDINGS
■ *Ability to open wide and close completely* Examine with eyes lightly closed, closed tightly, open wide.	**EXPECTED:** Superior eyelid covering a portion of iris when open. **UNEXPECTED:** Fasciculations when lightly closed. Ptosis. Lagophthalmos.
■ *Eyelid margin*	**UNEXPECTED:** Flakiness, redness, or swelling. Hordeola.
■ *Eyelashes*	**EXPECTED:** Present on both lids. Turned outward.
Palpate eyelids	
	UNEXPECTED: Nodules.
Palpate eye	
	EXPECTED: Can be gently pushed into orbit without discomfort. **UNEXPECTED:** Firm and resists palpation.

Pull down lower lids and inspect conjunctivae and sclerae

■ *Color* Inspect upper tarsal conjunctivae only if presence of foreign body is suspected.	**EXPECTED:** Conjunctivae clear and inapparent. Sclerae white and visible above irides only when eyelids are wide open. **UNEXPECTED:** Conjunctivae with erythema. Sclerae yellow or green. Sclerae with dark, rust-colored pigment anterior to insertion of medial rectus muscle.
■ *Condition*	**UNEXPECTED:** Exudate. Pterygium. Corneal arcus senilis or opacities.

Inspect lacrimal gland region

■ *Lacrimal gland puncta* Palpate lower orbital rim near inner canthus. If temporal aspect of upper lid feels full, evert lid and inspect gland.	**EXPECTED:** Slight elevations with central depression on both upper and lower lid margins. **UNEXPECTED:** Enlarged glands. Dry eyes.

TECHNIQUE	**FINDINGS**

Test corneal sensitivity

Touch wisp of cotton to cornea.

EXPECTED: Bilateral blink reflex.

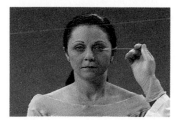

Inspect external eyes

- *Corneal clarity*
  Shine light tangentially on cornea.

UNEXPECTED: Blood vessels present.

- *Irides*

EXPECTED: Clearly visible pattern. Similar color.

- *Pupillary size/shape*

EXPECTED: Round, regular, equal in size.

UNEXPECTED: Miosis, mydriasis, anisocoria, or coloboma.

- *Pupillary response to light*

EXPECTED: Constricting with consensual response of opposite pupil.

- *Pupillary accommodation*

EXPECTED: Constricting when pupils focus on near object or dilating when focus changes from near to distant object.

- *Afferent pupillary testing*

EXPECTED: The pupil toward which the light is moving dilates and then constricts as the light shines onto it.

UNEXPECTED: The pupil continues to dilate when the light shines into it.

TECHNIQUE	FINDINGS

EXTRAOCULAR EYE MUSCLES

Evaluate muscle balance and movement of eyes

▪ *Six cardinal fields of gaze*
Hold patient's chin, and ask patient to watch finger or penlight.

EXPECTED: A few horizontal nystagmic beats. Smooth, full, coordinated movement of eyes.
UNEXPECTED: Sustained or jerking nystagmus. Exposure of sclera from lid lag. Inability of eye to move in all directions.

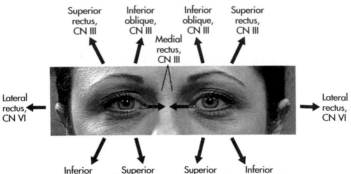

Superior rectus, CN III   Inferior oblique, CN III   Inferior oblique, CN III   Superior rectus, CN III

Medial rectus, CN III

Lateral rectus, CN VI   Lateral rectus, CN VI

Inferior rectus, CN III   Superior oblique, CN IV   Superior oblique, CN IV   Inferior rectus, CN III

▪ *Corneal light reflex*
Direct light at nasal bridge from 30 cm (12 inches). Have patient look at nearby object.

EXPECTED: Light reflected symmetrically from both eyes.

▪ *Cover-uncover test*
Perform if imbalance found with corneal light reflex test. Have patient stare ahead at near, fixed object. Cover one eye and observe other; remove cover and observe uncovered eye. Repeat with other eye.

UNEXPECTED: Movement of covered or uncovered eye.

TECHNIQUE	FINDINGS

OPHTHALMOSCOPIC EXAMINATION

Inspect internal eye

▓ *Lens clarity*
▓ *Anterior chamber*
Shine focused light tangentially at limbus. Note illumination of iris nasally.

UNEXPECTED: Shallow chamber. If observed, avoid mydriatics.

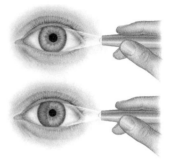

▓ *Use ophthalmoscope*
With patient looking at distant object, direct light at pupil from about 30 cm (12 inches). Move toward patient, observing:
▓ *Red reflex*
▓ *Fundus*

UNEXPECTED: Opacities.
EXPECTED: Yellow or pink background, depending on race. Possible crescents or dots of pigment at disc margin, usually temporally.
UNEXPECTED: Discrete areas of pigmentation away from disc. Lesions. Drusen bodies. Hemorrhages.

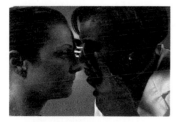

▓ *Blood vessel characteristics*
Follow blood vessels distally in each quadrant, noting crossings of arterioles and venules.

EXPECTED: Possible venous pulsations (should be documented). Arteriole/venule (A/V) ratio 3:5 or 2:3.
UNEXPECTED: Nicking, tortuosity.

TECHNIQUE **FINDINGS**

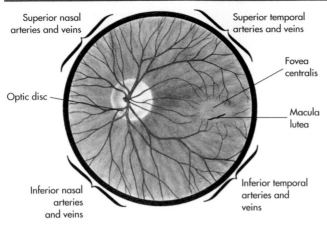

Superior nasal arteries and veins

Superior temporal arteries and veins

Fovea centralis

Optic disc

Macula lutea

Inferior nasal arteries and veins

Inferior temporal arteries and veins

■ *Disc characteristics*

EXPECTED: Yellow to creamy pink, varying by race. Sharp, well-defined margin, especially in temporal region; 1.5-mm diameter.
UNEXPECTED: Myelinated nerve fibers. Papilledema. Glaucomatous cupping.

■ *Macula densa characteristics*
Ask patient to look directly at light.

EXPECTED: Yellow dot surrounded by deep pink.

AIDS TO DIFFERENTIAL DIAGNOSIS

ABNORMALITY	DESCRIPTION
Strabismus (paralytic and nonparalytic)	Eyes cannot focus simultaneously. Can focus separately in nonparalytic type.
Episcleritis	Inflammation of superficial layers of sclera anterior to insertion of rectus muscles. Generally localized with purplish elevation of a few millimeters.
Cataracts	Opacity of lens, generally central, occasionally peripheral.

TECHNIQUE	FINDINGS
Diabetic retinopathy (background)	Dot hemorrhages or micro-aneurysms. Hard exudates (bright yellow, sharply defined borders) and soft exudates (dull yellow spots, poorly defined margins).
Proliferative	New vessel formation, extension out of the retina, hemorrhage.

PEDIATRIC VARIATIONS

EXAMINATION

TECHNIQUE	FINDINGS

VISUAL TESTING

Palpate superficial nodes

Measure visual acuity

■ *Distance vision*
Visual acuity is tested, when child is cooperative, with Lea cards, Landolt C or HOTV chart, usually at about 3 years of age.

EXPECTED:

Age, years	Acuity
3	20/50 or better
4	20/40 or better
5	20/30 or beter
6	20/20 or better

Infants should be able to focus on and track a face or light through 60 degrees.

EXTRAOCULAR EYE MUSCLES

Evaluate muscle balance and movement of eyes

Evaluation of six cardinal fields of gaze is performed as with adults. You may, however, need to hold child's head still.

SAMPLE DOCUMENTATION

Eyes. Near vision 20/40 in each eye uncorrected, corrected to 20/20 with glasses. Distant vision 20/20 by Snellen. Visual fields full by confrontation. Extraocular movements intact and full, no nystagmus. Corneal light reflex equal.

Lids and globes symmetric. No ptosis. Eyebrows full, no edema or lesions evident.

Conjunctivae pink, sclerae white. No discharge evident. Cornea clear, corneal reflex intact. Irides brown; pupils equal, round, reactive to light and accommodation.

Ophthalmoscopic examination reveals red reflex. Discs cream colored, borders well defined with temporal pigmentation in both eyes. No venous pulsations evident at disc. Arteriole/venule ratio 3:5; no nicking or crossing changes, hemorrhages, or exudates noted. Maculae are yellow in each eye.

Ears, Nose, and Throat

EQUIPMENT

- Otoscope with pneumatic attachment
- Tuning fork (500-1000 Hz)
- Nasal speculum
- Tongue blades
- Gloves
- Gauze
- Penlight, sinus transilluminator, or light from otoscope

EXAMINATION

Have patient sit.

TECHNIQUE	FINDINGS

EARS

Inspect auricles and mastoid area
Examine lateral and medial
surfaces and surrounding tissue.

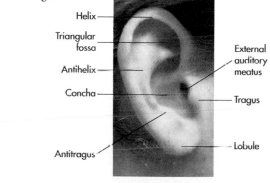

Helix
Triangular fossa
Antihelix
Concha
Antitragus
External auditory meatus
Tragus
Lobule

Auricle

TECHNIQUE	FINDINGS
■ *Size/shape/symmetry*	**EXPECTED:** Familial variations. Auricles of equal size and similar appearance. Darwin tubercle. **UNEXPECTED:** Unequal size or configuration. Cauliflower ear and other deformities.
■ *Lesions*	**UNEXPECTED:** Moles, cysts or other lesions, nodules, or tophi.
■ *Color*	**EXPECTED:** Same color as facial skin. **UNEXPECTED:** Blueness, pallor, or excessive redness.
■ *Position* Draw imaginary line between inner canthus and most prominent protuberance of occiput. Draw imaginary line perpendicular to first line and anterior to auricle.	**EXPECTED:** Top of auricle touching or above line. Vertical position. **UNEXPECTED:** Auricle positioned below line (low-set); unequal alignment. Lateral posterior angle greater than 10 degrees.
■ *Preauricular area*	**EXPECTED:** Preauricular pits or smooth skin. **UNEXPECTED:** Openings in preauricular area, discharge.
■ *External auditory canal*	**EXPECTED:** No discharge, no odor; canal walls pink. **UNEXPECTED:** Serous, bloody, or purulent discharge; foul smell.

Palpate auricles and mastoid area

EXPECTED: Firm and mobile, readily recoils from folded position; nontender.
UNEXPECTED: Tenderness, swelling, nodules. Pain from pulling on lobule.

Inspect auditory canal with otoscope

EXPECTED: Cerumen in varying color and texture.

TECHNIQUE	**FINDINGS**

Uniformly pink canal. Hairs in outer third of canal.
UNEXPECTED: Cerumen obscures tympanic membrane, odor, lesions, discharge, scaling, excessive redness, foreign bodies.

Inspect tympanic membrane

▪ *Landmarks*
Vary light direction to observe entire membrane and annulus.

EXPECTED: Visible landmarks (umbo, handle of malleus, light reflex).
UNEXPECTED: Perforations, landmarks not visible.

Chorda tympani nerve
12
Posterior malleolar folds
Pars flaccida
Junction of incus and stapes
Anterior malleolar folds
Short process of malleus
9
3
Manubrium (handle)
Pars tensa
Umbo
6
Light reflex

Tympanic membrane. *From Burkauskas et al, 2001.*

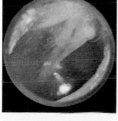

Tympanic membrane. *From Barkauskas et al, 2001.*

TECHNIQUE	FINDINGS
▨ *Color*	**EXPECTED:** Translucent, pearly gray. **UNEXPECTED:** Amber, yellow, blue, deep red, chalky white, dull, white flecks, or dense white plaques; air bubbles or fluid level.
▨ *Contour*	**EXPECTED:** Slightly conical with concavity at umbo. **UNEXPECTED:** Bulging (more conical, usually with loss of bony landmarks and distorted light reflex) or retracted (more concave, usually with accentuated bony landmarks and distorted light reflex).
▨ *Mobility* Seal canal with speculum, and gently apply positive (squeeze) and negative (release) pressure with pneumatic attachment.	**EXPECTED:** Movement in and out. **UNEXPECTED:** No movement.

Assess hearing

▨ *Questions during history*	**EXPECTED:** Responds to questions appropriately. **UNEXPECTED:** Excessive requests for repetition. Speech with monotonous tone and erratic volume.
▨ *Whispered voice* Have patient mask hearing in one ear by moving finger rapidly up and down in ear canal. Stand 1 to 2 feet from other ear and softly whisper three letter and number combinations (e.g., 3, T, 9 or 5, M, 2). Repeat with untested ear.	**EXPECTED:** Patient repeats words correctly more than 50% of the time. **UNEXPECTED:** Patient unable to repeat whispered words
▨ *Weber test* Place base of vibrating tuning fork on midline vertex of head. Repeat with one ear occluded.	**EXPECTED:** Sound heard equally in both ears (unoccluded). Sound heard better in occluded ear.

TECHNIQUE	**FINDINGS**

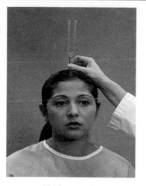

Weber test

UNEXPECTED: See table below.

■ *Rinne test*
Place base of vibrating tuning fork against mastoid bone, note seconds until sound is no longer heard; then quickly move fork 1 to 2 cm ($\frac{1}{2}$ to 1 inch) from auditory canal and note seconds until sound is no longer heard. Repeat with other ear.

EXPECTED: Measurement of air-conducted sound twice as long as measurement of bone-conducted sound.
UNEXPECTED: See table below.

Interpretation of Tuning Fork Tests

	Weber Test	Rinne Test
Expected findings	No lateralization but will lateralize to ear occluded by patient	Air conduction heard longer than bone conduction by 2:1 ratio (*Rinne positive*)
Conductive hearing loss	Lateralization to deaf ear unless sensorineural loss	Bone conduction heard longer than air conduction in affected ear (*Rinne negative*)
Sensorineural hearing loss	Lateralization to better-hearing ear unless conductive loss	Air conduction heard longer than bone conduction in affected ear, but less than 2:1 ratio

TECHNIQUE   **FINDINGS**

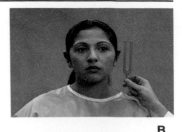

A   **B**

Rinne test. **A,** Tuning fork against mastoid bone. **B,** Tuning fork near ear.

NOSE AND SINUSES

Inspect external nose

■ *Shape/size*

EXPECTED: Smooth. Columella directly midline, width is not greater than diameter of naris.
UNEXPECTED: Swelling or depression of nasal bridge. Transverse crease at junction of nose cartilage and bone.

■ *Color*

EXPECTED: Conforms to face color.

■ *Nares*

EXPECTED: Oval. Symmetrically positioned
UNEXPECTED: Asymmetry, discharge, flaring, narrowing.

Palpate ridge and soft tissues of nose

Place one finger on each side of nasal arch and gently palpate from nasal bridge to tip.

EXPECTED: Firm and stable structures.
UNEXPECTED: Displacement of bone and cartilage, tenderness, or masses.

Evaluate patency of nares

Occlude one naris with finger on side of nose, ask patient to breathe through nose. Repeat with other naris.

EXPECTED: Noiseless, easy breathing.
UNEXPECTED: Noisy breathing; occlusion.

TECHNIQUE	FINDINGS

Inspect nasal mucosa and nasal septum

Tilt patient's head toward opposite shoulder. Pull auricle upward and back while gently inserting speculum. Assess canal from meatus to tympanic membrane.

■ *Color*

EXPECTED: Mucosa deep pink and glistening. Turbinates same color as surrounding area.

UNEXPECTED: Increased redness of mucosa or localized redness and swelling in vestibule. Turbinates bluish gray or pale pink.

■ *Shape*

EXPECTED: Septum close to midline and fairly straight, thicker anteriorly than posteriorly. Inferior and middle turbinates visible.

UNEXPECTED: Asymmetry of posterior nasal cavities, septal deviation.

■ *Condition*

EXPECTED: Possibly film of clear discharge on septum. Possibly hairs in vestibule. Turbinates firm.

UNEXPECTED: Discharge, bleeding, crusting, masses, or lesions. Swollen, boggy turbinates. Perforated septum. Polyps

SENSE OF SMELL

See Chapter 18.

TECHNIQUE	**FINDINGS**

Inspect frontal and maxillary sinus area

UNEXPECTED: Swelling.

Frontal sinuses
Ethmoid sinuses
Sphenoid sinus
Maxillary sinuses

Sinuses

Palpate frontal and maxillary sinuses

Press thumbs up under bony brow on each side of nose. Palpate with thumbs or index or middle fingers under zygomatic processes.

EXPECTED: Nontender on palpation.
UNEXPECTED: Tenderness or swelling.

MOUTH

Inspect and palpate lips with mouth closed

Have patient remove lipstick (if applicable).

■ *Symmetry*

EXPECTED: Symmetric vertically and horizontally at rest and while moving.
UNEXPECTED: Asymmetric.

■ *Color*

EXPECTED: Pink, distinct border between lips and facial skin.
UNEXPECTED: Pallor, circumoral pallor, bluish purple, or cherry red.

■ *Condition*

EXPECTED: Smooth.
UNEXPECTED: Dry, cracked; swelling, angioedema; cheilosis; lesions; plaques;

TECHNIQUE   **FINDINGS**

vesicles; nodules, ulcerations; or round, oval, or irregular bluish gray macules.

Inspect teeth

■ *Occlusion*

Have patient clench teeth and smile with lips spread.

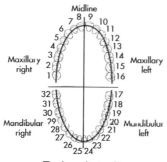

Teeth occlusion line

EXPECTED: Upper molars interdigitate with groove on lower molars. Premolars and canines interdigitate fully. Upper incisors slightly overriding lower incisors.
UNEXPECTED: Malocclusion. Protrusion of lower incisors. Problems with bite.

■ *Color*

EXPECTED: Ivory, stained yellow or brown.
UNEXPECTED: Discolorations may indicate caries.

■ *Condition*

EXPECTED: 32 teeth, firmly anchored.
UNEXPECTED: Caries and loose or missing teeth.

Inspect buccal mucosa

Have patient remove any dental appliances and then partially open mouth. Use tongue blade and bright light to assess.

■ *Color*

EXPECTED: Pinkish red.
UNEXPECTED: Deeply pigmented. Whitish or pinkish scars.

■ *Condition*

EXPECTED: Smooth and moist. Whitish yellow or whitish

TECHNIQUE	**FINDINGS**
	pink Stensen duct. Fordyce spots. **UNEXPECTED:** Adherent thickened white patch; white, round, or oval ulcerative lesions; red spot at opening of Stensen duct; stones or exudate from Stensen duct.

Inspect and palpate gingiva

Use gloves to palpate.

▨ *Color*	**EXPECTED:** Slightly stippled and pink. **UNEXPECTED:** Blue-black line about 1 mm from gum margin.
▨ *Condition*	**EXPECTED:** Clearly defined, tight margin at each tooth. **UNEXPECTED:** Inflammation, swelling, bleeding, or lesions under dentures or on gingiva; induration, thickening, masses, or tenderness. Enlarged crevices between teeth and gum margins. Pockets containing debris at tooth margins.

Inspect tongue

▨ *Size/symmetry*	**EXPECTED:** Midline, no fasciculations. **UNEXPECTED:** Atrophied, deviation to one side.
▨ *Color*	**EXPECTED:** Dull red.
▨ *Dorsum surface* Have patient extend tongue and hold extended.	**EXPECTED:** Moist and glistening. *Anterior:* Smooth yet roughened surface with papillae and small fissures. *Posterior:* Smooth, slightly uneven or rugated surface with thinner mucosa than anterior. Possibly geographic.

TECHNIQUE	FINDINGS

UNEXPECTED: Smooth, red, slick; hairy; swollen; coated; ulcerated; fasciculations; or limitation of movement.

■ *Ventral surface and floor of mouth*
Have patient touch tip of tongue to palate behind upper incisors.

EXPECTED: Ventral surface pink and smooth with large veins between frenulum and fimbriated folds. Wharton ducts apparent on each side of frenulum.
UNEXPECTED: Difficulty touching hard palate. Swelling, varicosities.

■ *Lateral borders*
Wrap tongue with gauze and pull to each side. Scrape white or red margins to remove food particles.

UNEXPECTED: Leukoplakia, ulceration, induration.

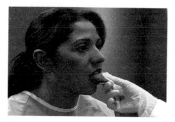

Inspecting lateral border of tongue

Palpate tongue and floor of mouth

EXPECTED: Smooth and even.
UNEXPECTED: Lumps, nodules, induration, ulcerations, or thickened white patches.

Inspect palate and uvula

Have patient tilt head back.
■ *Color and landmarks*

EXPECTED: Hard palate (whitish and dome-shaped with transverse rugae) contiguous with pinker soft palate. Bony protuberance of hard palate at midline (torus palatinus).
UNEXPECTED: Nodule on palate, not at midline.

TECHNIQUE	FINDINGS
■ *Movement* Ask patient to say "ah" while observing soft palate. (Depress tongue if necessary.)	**EXPECTED:** Soft palate rises symmetrically, with uvula remaining in midline. **UNEXPECTED:** Failure of soft palate to rise bilaterally. Uvula deviation. Bifid uvula.

Inspect oropharynx

Depress tongue with tongue blade.

■ *Tonsils* Inspect the tonsillar pillars and size of tonsils.	**EXPECTED:** Tonsils, if present, blend into pink color of pharynx. Possibly crypts in tonsils where cellular debris and food particles collect. **UNEXPECTED:** Tonsils projecting beyond limits of tonsillar pillars. Tonsils red, enlarged, covered with exudate.
■ *Posterior wall of pharynx*	**EXPECTED:** Smooth, glistening, pink mucosa with some small, irregular spots of lymphatic tissue and small blood vessels. **UNEXPECTED:** Red bulge adjacent to tonsil extending beyond midline. Yellowish mucoid film in pharynx. Grayish membrane.

Elicit gag reflex

Touch posterior wall of pharynx on each side	**EXPECTED:** Bilateral response. **UNEXPECTED:** Unequal response or no response.

AIDS TO DIFFERENTIAL DIAGNOSIS

ABNORMALITY	DESCRIPTION
Acute otitis media	See table on p. 90.
Middle ear effusion (serous otitis media)	See table on p. 90.

TECHNIQUE	FINDINGS
Sinusitis	Fever, headache, local tenderness, sinus pain or pressure, maxillary toothache, dull or opaque transillumination, nasal congestion, purulent nasal or postnasal discharge.
Tonsillitis	Sore throat, referred pain to ears, dysphagia, fever, fetid breath, malaise. Tonsils are red and swollen. Tonsils covered with purulent exudate. May be studded with yellow follicles. Enlarged anterior cervical lymph nodes.
Peritonsillar abscess	Dysphagia, drooling, severe sore throat with pain radiating to ear, muffled voice, fever. Tonsil, tonsillar pillar, adjacent soft palate are red and swollen. Tonsil may appear pushed forward or backward, possibly displacing uvula.
Oral cancer	Ulcerative lesion (red, white, pigmented) on lateral border of tongue, floor of mouth, gums, tonsil, or buccal mucosa; may be painless in early stage; may bleed; cervical adenopathy.
Periodontal disease	Easily bleeding, swollen gums, enlarged crevices between teeth and gum margins.
Malocclusion	Teeth malpositioned, upper and lower molars not aligned, line of occlusion is incorrect.
Dental caries	Discolorations on crown of tooth.

Differentiating Between Otitis Externa, Acute Otitis Media, and Middle Ear Effusion

Signs and Symptoms	Otitis Externa	Acute Otitis Media	Middle Ear Effusion
Initial symptoms	Itching in ear canal	Abrupt onset, fever, irritability, feeling of blockage	Sticking or cracking sound on yawning or swallowing; no signs of acute infection
Pain	Intense with movement of pinna or chewing	Deep-seated earache that interferes with activity or sleep, tugging at earlobe	Discomfort; feeling of fullness
Discharge	Watery, then purulent and thick mixed with pus and epithelial cells; musty, foul smelling	Only if tympanic membrane ruptures; foul smelling	Uncommon
Hearing	Conductive loss caused by exudate and swelling of ear canal	Conductive loss as middle ear fills with pus	Conductive loss as middle ear fills with fluid
Inspection	Canal is red, edematous, tympanic	Tympanic membrane with distinct erythema, thickened or clouding, bulging; limited movement to +/- pressure, air-fluid level, and/or bubbles	Tympanic membrane is retracted or bulging, yellowish; impaired mobility; visible air-fluid level and/or bubbles

PEDIATRIC VARIATIONS

EXAMINATION

TECHNIQUE	FINDINGS

EARS

Inspect tympanic membrane

In children, pull auricle downward and back.

EXPECTED: Tympanic membrane may be red from crying. If red from crying, it will be mobile.

Assess hearing

■ *Evaluate response to auditory stimuli (bell, clapped hands, tissue paper)*

EXPECTED: For infants, see table below. Young children should turn toward sound consistently.

Sequences of Expected Hearing and Speech Response in Infants

Age	Response
Birth to 3 months	Startle reflex, crying, cessation of breathing or movement in response to sudden noise; quiets to parent's voice; makes vowel sounds "oh" and "ah"
4 to 6 months	Turns head toward source of sound but may not always recognize location of sound; responds to parent's voice; enjoys sound-producing toys; starts babbling
6 to 10 months	Responds to own name, telephone ringing, and person's voice, even if not loud; begins localizing sounds above and below, turns head 45 degrees toward sound; babbles "baba," "mama," "gaga"; begins to imitate speech sounds
10 to 12 months	Recognizes and localizes source of sound; imitates simple words and sounds; understands "no-no" and "bye-bye"; correctly uses mama and dada

TECHNIQUE	FINDINGS

NOSE AND SINUSES

Evaluate patency of nares

With infant's mouth closed or with infant sucking on bottle or pacifier, occlude one naris and then the other. Observe respiratory pattern.

EXPECTED: Breathes easily; obligatory nose breathing until 2 to 3 months of age.

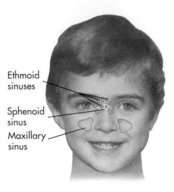

Ethmoid sinuses
Sphenoid sinus
Maxillary sinus

Pediatric sinuses

MOUTH

Inspect and palpate lips with mouth closed

EXPECTED: In infants aged 6 weeks to 6 months, sucking calluses, drooling.
UNEXPECTED: Drooling persistent after age 12 months.

Inspect teeth

■ *Color*

EXPECTED: 0 to 20 teeth until age 6 years. Permanent teeth start erupting around age 6 years.
UNEXPECTED: Natal teeth.

TECHNIQUE	FINDINGS
Inspect buccal mucosa	
■ *Condition*	**EXPECTED:** In infants, nonadherent white patches (milk). **UNEXPECTED:** In infants, adherent white patches.
Inspect and palpate gingiva	
■ *Condition*	**EXPECTED:** In infants, pearl-like retention cysts.

AIDS TO DIFFERENTIAL DIAGNOSIS

ABNORMALITY	DESCRIPTION
Cleft lip and palate	Fissure or cleft extending through upper lip or hard and soft palate into nasal cavity
Epiglottitis	High fever, croupy cough, sore throat, drooling, difficulty breathing.

SAMPLE DOCUMENTATION

Subjective. A 55-year-old man with concerns about hearing loss for the past few months, particularly with high-pitched tones. Has difficulty hearing on phone and in conversations when multiple people are talking. Hears "noise" in both ears when trying to go to sleep at night. No ear pain or discharge. No nasal discharge or sinus pain. No mouth lesions or masses; no recent dental problems; no sore throat.

Objective. *Ears:* Auricles in alignment. Canals totally obstructed by cerumen bilaterally. After irrigation, tympanic membranes are pearly gray, noninjected, intact, with bony landmarks and light reflex visualized bilaterally. No evidence of fluid or retraction. Conversational hearing appropriate. Able to hear whispered voice. Weber—lateralizes equally to both ears; Rinne—air conduction greater than bone conduction bilaterally (30 seconds/15 seconds). *Nose:* No discharge or polyps, mucosa pink and moist, septum midline, patent bilaterally. No edema over frontal or maxillary sinuses. No sinus tenderness to palpation. Correctly identifies mint, banana, ammonia odors. *Mouth:* Buccal mucosa pink and moist without lesions. Twenty-six teeth present in various states of repair. Lower second molars (18, 30) absent bilaterally. Gingiva pink and firm. Tongue midline with no tremors or fasciculation. Pharynx clear without erythema; tonsils 1+ without exudates. Uvula rises evenly, and gag reflex is intact. No hoarseness. Patient identifies tastes of salt and sugar.

EQUIPMENT

- Drape
- Skin-marking pencil
- Ruler and tape measure
- Stethoscope with bell and diaphragm

EXAMINATION

Have patient sit, disrobed to waist.

TECHNIQUE	FINDINGS

CHEST AND LUNGS

Inspect front and back of chest

See thoracic landmarks.

- *Size/shape/symmetry*
- *Landmarks*

EXPECTED: Supernumerary nipples possible (can be clue to other congenital abnormalities, particularly in whites).

- *Compare anteroposterior diameter with transverse diameter*

EXPECTED: Ribs prominent, clavicles prominent superiorly, sternum usually flat and free of abundance of overlying tissue. Chest somewhat asymmetric. Anteroposterior diameter often half of transverse diameter.

UNEXPECTED: Barrel chest, posterior or lateral deviation, pigeon chest, or funnel chest.

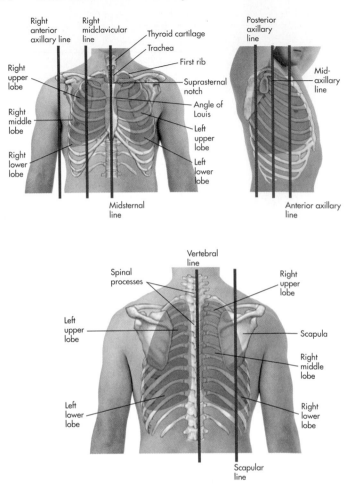

TECHNIQUE	FINDINGS
■ *Assess nails, lips, nares*	**UNEXPECTED:** Clubbed fingernails (usually symmetric and painless; may indicate disease, may be hereditary), pursed lips, flared alae nasi.
■ *Color* Assess skin, lips, nails.	**UNEXPECTED:** Superficial venous patterns. Cyanosis or pallor of lips or nails.
■ *Breath*	**UNEXPECTED:** Malodorous.

| **T E C H N I Q U E** | **F I N D I N G S** |

Evaluate respirations

■ *Rhythm or pattern and rate*
See patterns of respiration in
figure below.

EXPECTED: Breathing easy,
regular, without distress. Pattern
even. Rate 12 to 20 respirations
per minute. Ratio of respirations
to heartbeats about 1:4.
UNEXPECTED: Dyspnea,
orthopnea, paroxysmal
nocturnal dyspnea, platypnea,
tachypnea, hypopnea. Use of
accessory muscles, retractions.

Normal	Regular and comfortable at a rate of 12-20 per minute	Air trapping	Increasing difficulty in getting breath out
Bradypnea	Slower than 12 breaths per minute	Cheyne-Stokes	Varying periods of increasing depth interspersed with apnea
Tachypnea	Faster than 20 breaths per minute	Kussmaul	Rapid, deep, labored
Hyperventilation (hyperpnea)	Faster than 20 breaths per minute, deep breathing	Biot	Irregularly interspersed periods of apnea in a disorganized sequence of breaths
Sighing	Frequently interspersed deeper breath	Ataxic	Significant disorganization with irregular and varying depths of respiration

■ *Inspiration/expiration ratio*

UNEXPECTED: Air trapping,
prolonged expiration.

Inspect chest movement with breathing

■ *Symmetry*

EXPECTED: Chest expansion
bilaterally symmetric.
UNEXPECTED: Asymmetry.
Unilateral or bilateral bulging.
Bulging on expiration.

TECHNIQUE	FINDINGS

Listen to respiration sounds audible without stethoscope

EXPECTED: Generally bronchovesicular.
UNEXPECTED: Crepitus, stridor, wheezes.

Palpate thoracic muscles and skeleton

■ *Symmetry/condition*

EXPECTED: Bilateral symmetry. Some elasticity of rib cage, but sternum and xiphoid relatively inflexible and thoracic spine rigid.
UNEXPECTED: Pulsations, tenderness, bulges, depressions, unusual movement, unusual positions.

■ *Thoracic expansion*
Stand behind patient. Place palms in light contact with posterolateral surfaces and thumbs along spinal processes at tenth rib, as shown in figure at right. Watch thumb divergence during quiet and deep breathing. Face patient; place thumbs along costal margin and xiphoid process with palms touching anterolateral chest. Watch thumb divergence during quiet and deep breathing.

EXPECTED: Symmetric expansion.
UNEXPECTED: Asymmetric expansion.

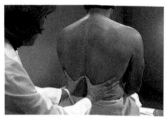

■ *Sensations*

EXPECTED: Nontender sensations.
UNEXPECTED: Crepitus or grating vibration.

TECHNIQUE	FINDINGS

■ *Tactile fremitus*
Ask patient to recite numbers or words while systematically palpating chest with palmar surfaces of fingers or ulnar aspect of clenched fist, using firm, light touch. Assess each area, front to back, side to side, lung apices. Compare sides.

EXPECTED: Great variability; generally, fremitus is more intense with males (lower-pitched voice).
UNEXPECTED: Decreased or absent fremitus; increased fremitus (coarser, rougher); or gentle, more tremulous fremitus. Variation between similar positions on right and left thorax.

Note position of trachea

Using index finger or thumbs, palpate gently from suprasternal notch along upper edges of each clavicle and in spaces above, to inner borders of sternocleidomastoid muscles.

EXPECTED: Spaces equal side to side. Trachea midline directly above suprasternal notch. Possible slight deviation to right.
UNEXPECTED: Significant deviation or tug. Pulsations.

Perform direct or indirect percussion on chest

Percuss directly or indirectly, as shown in figures below. Compare all areas bilaterally, following a sequence such as shown in figures on p. 100.
See table on p. 100 for common tones, intensity, pitch, duration, quality.

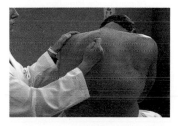
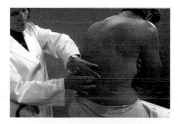

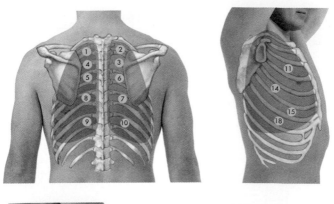

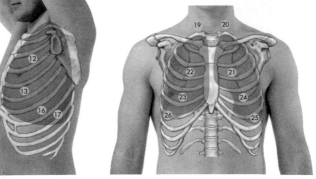

Percussion Tones Heard Over the Chest

Type of Tone	Intensity	Pitch	Duration	Quality
Resonant	Loud	Low	Long	Hollow
Flat	Soft	High	Short	Extremely dull
Dull	Medium	Medium-high	Medium	Thudlike
Tympanic	Loud	High	Medium	Drumlike
Hyperresonant*	Very loud	Very low	Longer	Booming

From Thompson et al, 1997.
*Hyperresonance is unexpected in adults. It represents air trapping, which occurs in obstructive lung diseases.

TECHNIQUE

■ *Thorax*
Have patient sit with head bent and arms folded in front while percussing posterior

FINDINGS

EXPECTED: Resonance over all areas of lungs, dull over heart and liver, spleen, areas of thorax.

TECHNIQUE	**FINDINGS**

thorax, then with arms raised overhead while percussing lateral and anterior chest. Percuss at 4- to 5-cm intervals over intercostal spaces, moving superior to inferior, medial to lateral. The female breast may obscure findings. You or the patient may need to shift the breast, but pay careful attention to modesty.

UNEXPECTED: Hyperresonance, dullness, or flatness.

■ *Diaphragmatic excursion*
Ask patient to breathe deeply and hold breath. Percuss along scapular line on one side until tone changes from resonant to dull. Mark skin. Allow patient to breathe normally, then repeat on other side. Have patient take several breaths, then exhale as much as possible and hold. On each side, percuss up from mark to change from dull to resonant. Tell patient to resume breathing comfortably. Measure excursion distance.

EXPECTED: 3 to 5 cm (higher on right than left).
UNEXPECTED: Limited descent.

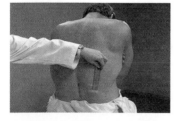

Auscultate chest with stethoscope diaphragm, apex to base

■ *Intensity, pitch, duration, and quality of breath sounds*
Have patient breathe slowly and deeply through mouth. Follow set auscultation

EXPECTED: See expected breath sounds in table on p. 102.
UNEXPECTED: Amphoric or cavernous breathing. Sounds difficult to hear or absent.

TECHNIQUE	FINDINGS
sequence, holding stethoscope as shown in figure at right. Ask patient to sit upright (1) with head bent and arms folded in front while auscultating posterior thorax, (2) with arms raised overhead while auscultating lateral chest, (3) with arms down and shoulders back while auscultating anterior chest.	Crackles, rhonchi, wheezes, or pleural friction rub, as described in box on p. 103.

Listen during inspiration and expiration. Auscultate downward from apex to base at intervals of several centimeters, making side-to-side comparisons.

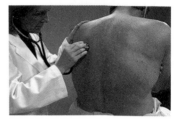

Characteristics of Expected Breath Sounds

Sound	Characteristics	Findings
Vesicular	Heard over most of lung fields; low pitch; soft and short expirations; will be accentuated in a thin person or a child and diminished in overweight or very muscular patient	
Bronchovesicular	Heard over main bronchus area and over upper right posterior lung field; medium pitch; expiration equals inspiration	
Bronchial tracheal (tubular)	Heard only over trachea; high pitch; loud and long expirations, often somewhat longer than inspiration	

Modified from Thompson et al, 1997.

Adventitious Breath Sounds

Fine crackles: High-pitched, discrete, discontinuous crackling sounds heard during end of inspiration; not cleared by cough

Medium crackles: Lower, more moist sound heard during midstage of inspiration; not cleared by cough

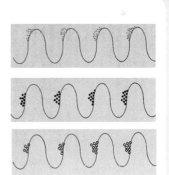

Coarse crackles: Loud, bubbly noise heard during inspiration; not cleared by cough

Rhonchi (sonorous wheeze): Loud, low, coarse sounds, like a snore, most often heard continuously during inspiration or expiration; coughing may clear sound (usually means mucus accumulation in trachea or large bronchi)

Wheeze (sibilant wheeze): Musical noise sounding like a squeak; most often heard continuously during inspiration or expiration; usually louder during expiration

Pleural friction rub: Dry rubbing or grating sound, usually caused by inflammation of pleural surfaces; heard during inspiration or expiration; loudest over lower lateral anterior surface

Modified from Thompson et al, 1997.

■ *Vocal resonance*
Ask patient to recite numbers or words.

EXPECTED: Muffled and indistinct sounds.
UNEXPECTED: Bronchophony, whispered pectoriloquy, or egophony.

AIDS TO DIFFERENTIAL DIAGNOSIS

ABNORMALITY	DESCRIPTION
Lung cancer	Cough, wheezing, emphysema, atelectasis, pneumonitis, hemoptysis. Possible sputum.
Infections	Sputum production (see table below).
Cough-producing conditions	See box on p. 105.
Asthma	Cough, wheezing, respiratory distress, tachypnea, pallor to cyanosis; possible decreased breath sounds; possibly allergy or exercise induced.
Chronic obstructive pulmonary disease	Barrel chest, hyperresonance to percussion, sputum production, cough, prolonged expiration, amphoric breathing.

Assessing Sputum

Cause	Possible Sputum Characteristics
Bacterial infection	Yellow, green, rust-colored (blood mixed with yellow sputum), clear, or transparent; purulent; blood streaked; mucoid, viscid
Viral infection	Mucoid, viscid; blood streaked (not common)
Chronic infectious disease	All of the above; particularly abundant in early morning; slight, intermittent blood streaking; occasionally large amounts of blood
Carcinoma	Slight, persistent blood streaking
Infarction	Blood clotted; large amounts of blood
Tuberculous cavity	Large amounts of blood

Assessing Cough

Coughs are common symptoms of a respiratory problem. They are usually preceded by a deep inspiration; this is followed by closure of the glottis, relaxation of the diaphragm, and then a sudden, spasmodic expiration, forcing a sudden opening of the glottis. Causes may be related to localized or more general insults at any point in the respiratory tract. Coughs may be voluntary, but they are usually reflexive responses to an irritant such as a foreign body (microscopic or larger), an infectious agent, or a mass of any sort compressing the respiratory tree. They may also be a clue to an anxiety state.

Describe a cough according to its moisture, frequency, regularity, pitch and loudness, and quality. The type of cough may offer some clue to the cause. Although a cough may not have a serious cause, it should not be ignored.

Dry or moist. A moist cough may be caused by infection and can be accompanied by sputum production. A dry cough can have a variety of causes (e.g., cardiac problems, allergies, or AIDS), which may be indicated by the quality of its sound.

Onset. Acute onset, particularly with fever, suggests infection; in the absence of fever, a foreign body or inhaled irritants are additional possible causes.

Frequency of occurrence. Note whether the cough is seldom or often present. Infrequent cough may result from allergens or environmental insults.

Regularity. A regular, paroxysmal cough is heard in pertussis. Irregularly occurring cough may have a variety of causes, such as smoking, early congestive heart failure, an inspired foreign body or irritant, or a tumor within or compressing the bronchial tree.

Pitch and loudness. A cough may be loud and high-pitched or quiet and relatively low-pitched.

Postural influences. A cough may occur soon after a person has reclined or assumed an erect position (e.g., with a nasal drip or pooling of secretions in the upper airway).

Quality. A dry cough may sound brassy if it is caused by compression of the respiratory tree (as by a tumor) or hoarse if it is caused by croup. Pertussis produces an inspiratory "whoop" at the end of a paroxysm of coughing.

PEDIATRIC VARIATIONS

EXAMINATION

TECHNIQUE **FINDINGS**

CHEST AND LUNGS

Inspect front and back of chest

- *Compare anteroposterior diameter with transverse diameter*

EXPECTED: Infant's chest is expected to measure 2 to 3 cm less than head circumference.

Evaluate respirations

- *Rhythm or pattern and rate*

EXPECTED:

Age	Respirations per minute
Newborn	30-80
1 year	20-40
3 years	20-30
6 years	16-22
10 years	16-20
17 years	12-20

Perform direct or indirect percussion on chest

- *Thorax*

EXPECTED: Hyperresonance may be heard in children.

Auscultate chest with stethoscope diaphragm, apex to base

- *Intensity, pitch, duration, and quality of breath sounds*

EXPECTED: In infants and children, expect transmitted breath sounds throughout chest. Vesicular sound will be accentuated in a child. Absent or diminished breath sounds are harder to detect.

SAMPLE DOCUMENTATION

Subjective. A 45-year-old woman complaining of cough and fever for 4 days. Cough is nonproductive, persistent, and worse when she lies down. She feels ill and short of breath. Her chest feels "heavy." Fever up to 38.3° C (101° F). Taking acetaminophen and nonprescription cough syrup without relief.

Objective. Minimal increase in anteroposterior diameter of chest, without kyphosis or other defect. Trachea in midline without tug. Thoracic expansion symmetric. Respirations 32 per minute and somewhat labored; no retractions or stridor. No friction rubs or tenderness over ribs or other bony prominences. Over posterior left base, diminished tactile fremitus, dull percussion note, and on auscultation, crackles that do not clear with cough, diminished breath sounds. Remaining lung fields are clear and free of adventitious sounds, with resonant percussion tones. Diaphragmatic excursion 3 cm bilaterally.

NOTE: Expected abnormal findings, as with pneumonia, may not be present consistently. Flaring of the alae nasi, tachypnea, and cough, particularly productive cough, may signal pneumonia even in the absence of crackles.

EQUIPMENT

- Tangential light source
- Skin-marking pencil
- Stethoscope with bell and diaphragm
- Centimeter ruler

EXAMINATION

TECHNIQUE   **FINDINGS**

HEART

Inspect precordium

Have patient supine, and keep
light source tangential.
- *Apical impulse*

EXPECTED: Visible about
midclavicular line in fifth left
intercostal space. Sometimes
visible only with patient sitting.
UNEXPECTED: Visible in
more than one intercostal space;
exaggerated lifts or heaves.

Palpate precordium

- *Apical impulse*
  Have patient supine. With
  hands *warm,* gently feel
  precordium, using proximal
  halves of fingers held together
  or whole hand. As shown in
  figure on p. 109, methodically
  move from apex to left sternal
  border, base, right sternal
  border, epigastrium, axillae.

EXPECTED: Gentle, brief
impulse, palpable within radius
of 1 cm or less, although often
not felt.
UNEXPECTED: Heave or lift,
loss of thrust, displacement to
right or left; thrill.

TECHNIQUE	FINDINGS

Locate sensation in terms of its intercostal space and relationship to midsternal, midclavicular, axillary lines.

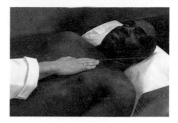

Percuss precordium (optional)

Begin by tapping at anterior axillary line, moving medially along intercostal spaces toward sternal borders until tone changes from resonance to dullness. Mark skin with pencil.

EXPECTED: No change in tone before right sternal border; on left, loss of resonance generally close to point of maximal impulse at fifth intercostal space. Loss of resonance may outline left border of heart at second to fifth intercostal spaces.

Auscultate heart

Make certain patient is warm and relaxed. Isolate each sound and each pause in cycle, and then inch along with stethoscope. Approach each of the five precordial areas shown in figure below systematically, base to apex or apex to base, using each position shown in figures at right. Use diaphragm of stethoscope first, with firm pressure, then bell, with light pressure.

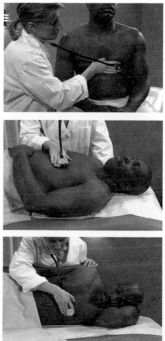

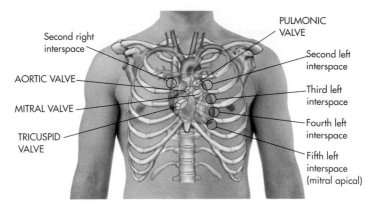

Second right interspace

PULMONIC VALVE

AORTIC VALVE

Second left interspace

MITRAL VALVE

Third left interspace

TRICUSPID VALVE

Fourth left interspace

Fifth left interspace (mitral apical)

TECHNIQUE	FINDINGS
■ *Rate and rhythm* Assess overall rate and rhythm.	**EXPECTED:** Rate 60 to 90 beats per minute, regular rhythm. **UNEXPECTED:** Bradycardia, tachycardia, arrhythmia.
■ S_1 Ask patient to breathe comfortably, then hold breath in expiration. Listen for S_1 (best heard toward apex) while palpating carotid pulse. Note intensity, variations, effect of respiration, splitting. Concentrate on systole, then diastole.	**EXPECTED:** S_1 usually heard as one sound and coincides with rise of carotid pulse. See table on p. 111 and figure on p. 113. **UNEXPECTED:** Extra sounds or murmurs.
■ S_2 Ask patient to breathe comfortably as you listen for S_2 (best heard in aortic and pulmonic areas) to become two components during inspiration. Ask patient to inhale and hold breath.	**EXPECTED:** S_2 to become two components during inspiration. S_2 to become an apparent single sound as breath is exhaled. See table on p. 111 and figure on p. 113.
■ *Splitting*	**EXPECTED:** S_2 splitting— greatest at peak of inspiration— varying from easily heard to nondetectable.

Heart Sounds According to Auscultatory Area

	Aortic	Pulmonic	Second Pulmonic	Mitral	Tricuspid
Pitch	$S_1 < S_2$	$S_1 < S_2$	$S_1 < S_2$	$S_1 > S_2$	$S_1 = S_2$
Loudness	$S_1 < S_2$	$S_1 < S_2$	$S_1 < S_2$*	$S_1 > S_2$†	$S_1 > S_2$
Duration	$S_1 < S_2$	$S_1 > S_2$	$S_1 < S_2$	$S_1 < S_2$	$S_1 = S_2$
S_2 split	>Inhale	>Inhale	>Inhale	>Inhale‡	>Inhale
	<Exhale	<Exhale	<Exhale	<Exhale	<Exhale
A_2	Loudest	Loud	Decreased		
P_2	Decreased	Louder	Loudest		

*S_1 is relatively louder in second pulmonic area than in aortic area.
†S_1 may be louder in mitral area than in tricuspid area.
‡S_2 split may not be audible in mitral area if P_2 is inaudible.

TECHNIQUE

■ S_3 and S_4
If needed, ask patient to raise a leg to increase venous return or to grip your hand vigorously and repeatedly to increase venous return.

■ *Extra heart sounds*

FINDINGS

EXPECTED: Both S_3 and S_4 quiet and difficult to hear. S_3 has rhythm of Ken-tuc-ky; S_4, Tenn-es-see.

UNEXPECTED: Increased intensity (and ease of hearing) of either.

UNEXPECTED: Extra heart sounds—snaps, clicks, friction rubs, murmurs. See table on p. 112 and figure on p. 113

Assess characteristics of murmurs

■ *Timing and duration, pitch, intensity, pattern, quality, location, radiation, respiratory phase variations*

Extra Heart Sounds

Sound	Detection	Description
Increased S_3	Bell at apex; patient left lateral recumbent	Early diastole, low pitch
Increased S_4	Bell apex; patient supine or semilateral	Late diastole or early systole, low pitch
Gallops	Bell at apex; patient supine or left lateral recumbent	Presystole, intense, easily heard
Mitral valve opening snap	Diaphragm medial to apex, may radiate to base; any position, second left intercostal	Early diastole briefly, before S_3; high pitch, sharp snap or click; not affected by respiration; easily confused with S_2
Ejection clicks	Diaphragm; patient sitting or supine	
Aortic valve	Apex, base in second intercostal space	Early systole, intense, high pitch; radiates, not affected by respirations
Pulmonary valve	Second left intercostal right space at sternal border	Early systole, less intense than aortic click; intensifies on expiration, decreases on inspiration
Pericardial friction rub	Widely heard, sound clearest toward apex	May occupy all of systole and diastole; intense, grating, machinelike; may have three components and obliterate heart sounds; if only one or two components, may sound like murmur

Heart sounds

Site at which best heard

Intense first sound	S_1 S_2	Apex
Split first sound	S_1 M T S_2	Tricuspid
Intense second sound	S_2 S_1	Base
Physiologic splitting—S_2 Expiration	S_2 S_1	Base
Inspiration	S_1 S_2 A P	
Third sound (ventricular gallop)	S_1 S_2 S_3	Apex
Fourth sound (atrial gallop)	S_4 S_1 S_2	Apex
Summation gallop	S_1 S_2 S_{3-4}	Apex

AIDS TO DIFFERENTIAL DIAGNOSIS

ABNORMALITY	DESCRIPTION
Chest pain	See table below.
Left ventricular hypertrophy	Vigorous sustained lift palpable during ventricular systole, sometimes over broader area than usual (by 2 cm or more). Displacement of apical impulse can be well lateral of midclavicular line and downward.
Right ventricular hypertrophy	Lift along left sternal border in third and fourth left intercostal spaces accompanied by occasional systolic retraction at apex. Left

Chest Pain

Type of Chest Pain	Characteristics
Anginal	Substernal; provoked by effort, emotion, eating; relieved by rest and/or nitroglycerin
Pleural	Precipitated by breathing or coughing; usually described as sharp
Esophageal	Burning, substernal, occasional radiation to shoulder; nocturnal occurrence, usually when lying flat; relief with food, antacids, sometimes nitroglycerin
From a peptic ulcer	Almost always infradiaphragmatic and epigastric; nocturnal occurrence and daytime attacks; should not be relieved by food; unrelated to activity
Biliary	Usually under right scapula, prolonged in duration; will trigger angina more often than mimic it
From arthritis/bursitis	Usually of hours-long duration; local tenderness and/or pain with movement
Cervical	Associated with injury; provoked by activity, persists after activity; painful on palpation and/or movement
Musculoskeletal (chest)	Intensified or provoked by movement, particularly twisting or costochondral bending; long-lasting; often associated with local tenderness
Psychoneurotic	Associated with or occurring after anxiety; poorly described, located in intramammary region

Data from Samiy et al, 1987; Harvey et al, 1988.

ABNORMALITY	DESCRIPTION
	ventricle displaced and turned posteriorly by enlarged right ventricle.
Congestive heart failure	Congestion in pulmonary or systemic circulation. Can be predominantly left- or right-sided and can develop gradually or suddenly with acute pulmonary edema.
Cor pulmonale	Left parasternal systolic lift and loud S_2 in pulmonic region.
Myocardial infarction	Deep substernal or visceral pain, often radiating to jaw, neck, left arm (although discomfort is sometimes mild); women may experience milder and different symptoms; dysrhythmias; S_4 often present. Heart sounds distant, with soft, systolic, blowing murmur; pulse possibly thready; varied blood pressure (although hypertension usual in early phases).
Myocarditis	*Initial:* Fatigue, dyspnea, fever, palpitations. *Later:* Cardiac enlargement, murmur, gallop rhythms, tachycardia, dysrhythmias, pulsus alternans.
Conduction disturbances	Transient weakness, fainting spells, or strokelike episodes.
Atherosclerotic heart disease	May cause myocardial insufficiency, angina pectoris, dysrhythmias, congestive heart failure.
Angina	Substernal pain or intense pressure radiating at times to neck, jaws, arms, particularly left arm. Often accompanied by shortness of breath, fatigue, diaphoresis, faintness, syncope. Cessation of activity may relieve pain.

PEDIATRIC VARIATIONS

EXAMINATION

TECHNIQUE	FINDINGS
Assess characteristics of murmurs	
▪ *Timing and duration, intensity, pattern, quality, location, radiation, respiratory phase variations*	In children it is necessary to distinguish innocent murmurs from organic murmurs caused by congenital defect or rheumatic fever.

AIDS TO DIFFERENTIAL DIAGNOSIS

ABNORMALITY	DESCRIPTION
Chest pain	Unlike in adults, chest pain in children and adolescents is seldom caused by a cardiac problem. It is very often difficult to find a cause, but trauma and exercise-induced asthma and use of cocaine, even in a somewhat younger child, as in the adolescent and adult, should be among the considerations.
Congenital defects	
Tetralogy of Fallot	Parasternal heave and precordial prominence. Cyanosis. Systolic ejection murmur heard over third intercostal space, sometimes radiating to left side of neck. Single S_2.
Ventricular septal defect	Arterial pulse small, and jugular venous pulse unaffected. Regurgitation occurs through septal defect, resulting in holosystolic murmur that is frequently loud, coarse, high-pitched, best heard along left sternal border in third to fifth intercostal spaces. Distinct lift

ABNORMALITY	DESCRIPTION
	often discernible along left sternal border and apical area. Does not radiate to neck.
Patent ductus arteriosus	Neck vessels dilated and pulsate, and pulse pressure wide. Harsh, loud, continuous murmur with machinelike quality, heard at first to third intercostal spaces and lower sternal border. Murmur usually unaltered by postural change.
Atrial septal defect	Systolic ejection murmur— best heard over pulmonic area—that is diamond-shaped, often loud, high in pitch, and harsh. May be accompanied by brief, rumbling, early diastolic murmur. Does not usually radiate beyond precordium. Systolic thrill may be felt over area of murmur along with palpable parasternal thrust. S_2 may be split fairly widely. Particularly significant with palpable thrust and occasional radiation through to back.
Dextrocardia and situs inversus	Altered clinical manifestations of disease (e.g., substernal pressure of myocardial ischemia) may be felt to right of precordium and may more often radiate to right arm.

SAMPLE DOCUMENTATION

Heart. No visible pulsations over precordium. Point of maximal impulse (PMI) palpable at the fifth ICS in the MCL, 1 cm in diameter. No lifts, heaves, or thrills felt on palpation. S_1 is crisp. Split S_2 increases with inspiration. No audible S_3, S_4, murmur, click, or rub.

EQUIPMENT

- Tangential light source
- Stethoscope with bell and diaphragm
- Sphygmomanometer
- Centimeter ruler

EXAMINATION

TECHNIQUE	FINDINGS

PERIPHERAL ARTERIES

Palpate arterial pulses in neck and extremities

Palpate carotid, brachial, radial, femoral, popliteal, dorsalis pedis, and posterior tibial arteries, using distal pads of second and third fingers, as shown in figures below and on p. 119.

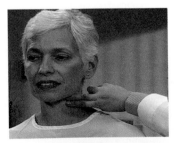

Carotid

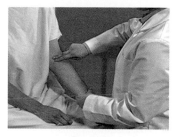

Brachial

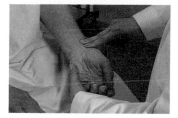

Radial

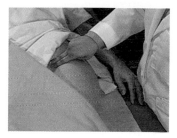

Femoral

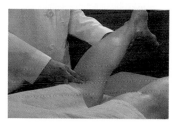

Popliteal

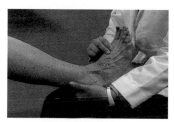

Dorsalis pedis

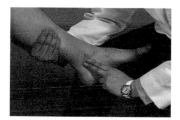

Posterior tibial

TECHNIQUE

■ *Characteristics*
Compare characteristics
bilaterally, as well as between
upper and lower extremities.

FINDINGS

EXPECTED: Femoral pulse as
strong as or stronger than radial
pulse.
UNEXPECTED: Femoral
pulse weaker than radial pulse or
absent. Alternating pulse (pulsus
alternans), pulsus bisferiens,
bigeminal pulse (pulsus
bigeminus), bounding pulse,
labile pulse, paradoxic pulse
(pulsus paradoxus), pulsus
differens, tachycardia, trigeminal

TECHNIQUE	FINDINGS
	pulse (pulsus trigeminus), or water-hammer pulse (Corrigan pulse).
▧ *Rate*	**EXPECTED:** 60 to 90 beats per minute. **UNEXPECTED:** Rate different from that observed during cardiac examination.
▧ *Rhythm*	**EXPECTED:** Regular. **UNEXPECTED:** Irregular, either in a pattern or patternless.
▧ *Contour*	**EXPECTED:** Smooth, rounded, or dome shaped.
▧ *Amplitude*	**UNEXPECTED:** Bounding, full, diminished, or absent. Describe on scale of 0 to 4: 0 = Absent, not palpable 1 = Diminished 2 = Expected 3 = Full, increased 4 = Bounding

Auscultate temporal, carotid, and subclavian arteries; abdominal aorta; and renal, iliac, and femoral arteries for bruits

When auscultating the carotid vessels, you may at times need to ask patient to hold breath for a few heartbeats. Auscultate with bell of stethoscope.	**UNEXPECTED:** Transmitted murmurs, bruits.

Assess for arterial occlusion and insufficiency

▧ *Site* Assess for pain distal to possible occlusion.	**UNEXPECTED:** Dull ache accompanied by fatigue and often crampiness; possible constant or excruciating pain. Weak, thready, or absent pulses; systolic bruits over arteries; loss of body warmth; localized pallor or cyanosis; delay in venous filling; or thin, atrophied skin, muscle atrophy, and loss of hair.

TECHNIQUE	FINDINGS
■ *Degree of occlusion* Ask patient to lie supine. Elevate extremity, note degree of blanching, then ask patient to sit on edge of table or bed to lower extremity. Note time for maximal return of color when extremity is lowered.	**EXPECTED:** Slight pallor on elevation and return to full color as soon as leg becomes dependent. **UNEXPECTED:** Delay of more than 2 seconds.
Measure blood pressure Measure in both arms at least once. Patient's arm should be slightly flexed and comfortably supported on table, pillow, or your hand.	**EXPECTED:** 100 to 140 mm Hg systolic and 60 to 90 mm Hg second diastolic, with pulse pressure of 30 to 40 mm Hg (sometimes to 50 mm Hg). Reading between arms may vary by as much as 10 mm Hg; usually higher in right arm. Prehypertension is now defined as a blood pressure

Classification of Blood Pressure for Adults Age 18 Years and Older*

Category	Systolic (mm Hg)		Diastolic (mm Hg)
Optimal[†]	<120	and	<80
Prehypertension	120-139	or	80-89
Hypertension[‡]			
Stage 1	140-159	or	90-99
Stage 2	160-179	or	100-109
Stage 3	≥180	or	≥110

From NIH Publication No. 4-5230, 2003.

*Not taking antihypertensive drugs and not acutely ill. When systolic and diastolic blood pressures fall into different categories, the higher category should be selected to classify the individual's blood pressure status. For example, 160/92 mm Hg should be classified as stage 2 hypertension, and 124/120 mm Hg should be classified as stage 3 hypertension. Isolated systolic hypertension is defined as systolic blood pressure of 140 mm Hg or greater and diastolic blood pressure below 90 mm Hg and staged appropriately (e.g., 170/82 mm Hg is defined as stage 2 isolated systolic hypertension). In addition to classifying stages of hypertension on the basis of average blood pressure levels, clinicians should specify presence or absence of target organ disease and additional risk factors. Specificity is important for risk classification and treatment.

†Optimal blood pressure with respect to cardiovascular risk is below 120/80 mm Hg. However, unusually low readings should be evaluated for clinical significance.

†Based on the average of two or more readings taken at each of two or more visits after an initial screening.

TECHNIQUE	FINDINGS

between 120 and 139 mm Hg systolic or 80 and 89 mm Hg diastolic.
UNEXPECTED: Hypertension (see table on p. 121).

PERIPHERAL VEINS

Assess jugular venous pressure

Ask patient to recline at 45-degree angle. With tangential light, observe both jugular veins. As shown in figure below, use a centimeter ruler to measure vertical distance between midaxillary line and highest level of jugular vein distention.

EXPECTED: Pressure 9 cm H_2O or less, bilaterally symmetric.
UNEXPECTED: Abnormal elevation, distention or distention on one side.

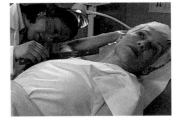

Assess for venous obstruction and insufficiency

Inspect extremities, with patient both standing and supine.

■ *Affected area*

UNEXPECTED: Constant pain with swelling and tenderness over muscles, engorgement of superficial veins, cyanosis.

■ *Thrombosis*
Flex patient's knee slightly with one hand, and with other, dorsiflex foot to test for Homans sign.

UNEXPECTED: Redness, thickening, tenderness along superficial vein. Calf pain with test for Homans sign.

■ *Edema*
Press index finger over bony

UNEXPECTED: Orthostatic (pitting) edema; thickening and

TECHNIQUE	**FINDINGS**
prominence of tibia or medial malleolus for several seconds.	ulceration of skin possible. Grade edema from 1+ to 4+ as follows: 1+ = Slight pitting, no visible distortion, disappears rapidly 2+ = Deeper than 1+ and disappears in 10 to 15 seconds 3+ = Noticeably deep and may last more than 1 minute, with dependent extremity full and swollen 4+ = Very deep and lasts 2 to 5 minutes, with grossly distorted dependent extremity
▪ *Varicose veins* If suspected, have patient stand on toes 10 times in succession.	**EXPECTED:** Pressure from toe standing disappears in seconds. **UNEXPECTED:** Veins dilated and swollen; often tortuous when extremities are dependent and pressure does not quickly disappear.
If varicose veins are present, assess venous incompetence with Trendelenburg test: Ask patient to lie supine, lift leg above heart level until veins empty, then quickly lower leg.	**UNEXPECTED:** Rapid filling of veins.
Evaluate patency of deep veins with Perthes test: Ask patient to lie supine. Elevate extremity, and occlude subcutaneous veins with tourniquet just above knee. Then ask patient to walk.	**UNEXPECTED:** Superficial veins fail to empty.
Evaluate direction of blood flow and presence of compensatory circulation: Put affected limb in dependent position, then empty or strip vein. Release	**UNEXPECTED:** Stripped vessel fills before pressure is released by distal finger, or blood refills entire vein when pressure is released by proximal finger.

TECHNIQUE	FINDINGS
pressure of one finger nearest heart to assess blood flow; if necessary, repeat and release pressure of other finger.	

AIDS TO DIFFERENTIAL DIAGNOSIS

ABNORMALITY	DESCRIPTION
Arterial aneurysm	Pulsatile dilatation along course of an artery—most commonly in the aorta, although intracranial, renal, femoral, and popliteal arteries are also affected. Thrill or bruit sometimes evident over aneurysm.
Venous thrombosis	Clinical findings in superficial vein include redness, thickening, tenderness along involved segment. Deep vein thrombosis in femoral and pelvic circulations may be asymptomatic, but suggestive signs and symptoms include tenderness along iliac vessels and femoral canal, in popliteal space, and over deep calf veins, as well as slight swelling, minimal ankle edema, low-grade fever, and tachycardia.
Raynaud disease	Intermittent skin pallor followed by cyanosis, bilateral and lasting from minutes to hours. Skin over digits eventually appears smooth, shiny, tight; ulcers may appear on tips of digits.

PEDIATRIC VARIATIONS

TECHNIQUE	FINDINGS

Palpate arterial pulses in distal extremities

■ *Rate*

EXPECTED:

Age	Beats per minute
Newborn	120-170
1 year	80-160
3 years	80-120
6 years	75-115
10 years	70-110

Auscultate arteries for bruits

EXPECTED: In children it is not unusual to hear a venous hum over internal jugular veins. There is usually no pathologic significance.

Measure blood pressure

When measuring an infant's blood pressure, use flush technique if needed.

EXPECTED: Calculation of systolic blood pressure for children older than 1 year can be estimated with following formula:

80 + (2 × Child's age in years)

Example: Calculation of expected systolic blood pressure of 5-year-old child:

80 + (2 × 5) = 90

Although this calculation gives a figure below the expected mean, it is still considered within normal limits for a 5-year-old child.

UNEXPECTED: Hypertension (see tables on pp. 127-130).

AIDS TO DIFFERENTIAL DIAGNOSIS

ABNORMALITY	DESCRIPTION
Coarctation of the aorta	Delay and/or palpable diminution in amplitude (not necessarily an absence) of femoral pulse when radial and femoral pulses are palpated simultaneously. Findings are same on right and left sides. Blood pressure in arms will be distinctly, even dramatically, higher than in legs. Possible systolic murmur audible over precordium and sometimes over back relative to area of coarctation. Adult x-ray examination may show notching of ribs and "3" sign in contour of left upper border of heart.

SAMPLE DOCUMENTATION

Vessels. Neck veins not distended. Both A and V waves are visualized. Jugular venous pressure (JVP) is 4 cm water at 45 degrees. Arterial pulses equal and symmetric, testing on a scale of 1/4.

	C	B	R	F	P	PT	DP
L	2 +	2 +	2 +	2 +	2 +	2 +	2 +
R	2 +	2 +	2 +	2 +	2 +	2 +	2 +

Vessels soft. No bruits are audible.

Extremities. No edema, skin, or nail changes. Superficial varicosities noted in both lower extremities. No areas of tenderness to palpation.

Blood Pressure Levels for the 90th and 95th Percentiles of Blood Pressure for Boys Age 1 to 17 Years by Percentiles of Height

Age, Years	Blood Pressure Percentile*	Systolic Blood Pressure by Percentile of Height, mm Hg†							Diastolic Blood Pressure by Percentile of Height, mm Hg†						
		5th	10th	25th	50th	75th	90th	95th	5th	10th	25th	50th	75th	90th	95th
1	90th	94	95	97	99	100	102	103	49	50	51	52	53	53	54
	95th	98	99	101	103	104	106	106	54	54	55	56	57	58	58
2	90th	97	99	100	102	104	105	106	54	55	56	57	58	58	59
	95th	101	102	104	106	108	109	110	59	59	60	61	62	63	63
3	90th	100	101	103	105	107	108	109	59	59	60	61	62	63	63
	95th	104	105	107	109	110	112	113	63	63	64	65	66	67	67
4	90th	102	103	105	107	109	110	111	62	63	64	65	66	66	67
	95th	106	107	109	111	112	114	115	66	67	68	69	70	71	71
5	90th	104	105	106	108	110	111	112	65	66	67	68	69	69	70
	95th	108	109	110	112	114	115	116	69	70	71	72	73	74	74
6	90th	105	106	108	110	111	113	113	68	68	69	70	71	72	72
	95th	109	110	112	114	115	117	117	72	72	73	74	75	76	76
7	90th	106	107	109	111	113	114	115	70	70	71	72	73	74	74
	95th	110	111	113	115	117	118	119	74	74	75	76	77	78	78
8	90th	107	109	110	112	114	115	116	71	72	72	73	74	75	76
	95th	111	112	114	116	118	119	120	75	76	77	78	79	79	80

Continued

From The Fourth Report on the Diagnosis, Evaluation, and Treatment of High Blood Pressure in Children and Adolescents, 2004.
*Blood pressure percentile was determined by a single measurement.
†Height percentile was determined by standard growth curves.

Blood Pressure Levels for the 90th and 95th Percentiles of Blood Pressure for Boys Age 1 to 17 Years by Percentiles of Height—cont'd

Age, Years	Blood Pressure Percentile*	Systolic Blood Pressure by Percentile of Height, mm Hg†							Diastolic Blood Pressure by Percentile of Height, mm Hg†						
		5th	10th	25th	50th	75th	90th	95th	5th	10th	25th	50th	75th	90th	95th
9	90th	109	110	112	114	115	117	117	72	73	74	75	76	76	77
	95th	113	114	116	118	119	121	121	76	77	78	79	80	81	81
10	90th	111	112	114	115	117	119	119	73	73	74	75	76	77	78
	95th	115	116	117	119	121	122	123	77	78	79	80	81	81	82
11	90th	113	114	115	117	119	120	121	74	74	75	76	77	78	78
	95th	117	118	119	121	123	124	125	78	78	79	80	81	82	82
12	90th	115	116	118	120	121	123	123	74	75	75	76	77	78	79
	95th	119	120	122	123	125	127	127	78	79	80	81	82	82	83
13	90th	117	118	120	122	124	125	126	75	75	76	77	78	79	79
	95th	121	122	124	126	128	129	130	79	79	80	81	82	83	83
14	90th	120	121	123	125	126	128	128	75	76	77	78	79	79	80
	95th	124	125	127	128	130	132	132	80	80	81	82	83	84	84
15	90th	122	124	125	127	129	130	131	76	77	78	79	80	80	81
	95th	126	127	129	131	133	134	135	81	81	82	83	84	85	85
16	90th	125	126	128	130	131	133	134	78	78	79	80	81	82	82
	95th	129	130	132	134	135	137	137	82	83	83	84	85	86	87
17	90th	127	128	130	132	134	135	136	80	80	81	82	83	84	84
	95th	131	132	134	136	138	139	140	84	85	86	87	87	88	89

From The Fourth Report on the Diagnosis, Evaluation, and Treatment of High Blood Pressure in Children and Adolescents, 2004.
*Blood pressure percentile was determined by a single measurement.
†Height percentile was determined by standard growth curves.

Blood Pressure Levels for the 90th and 95th Percentiles of Blood Pressure for Girls Age 1 to 17 Years by Percentiles of Height

Age, Years	Blood Pressure Percentile*	Systolic Blood Pressure by Percentile of Height†, mm Hg							Diastolic Blood Pressure by Percentile of Height†, mm Hg						
		5th	10th	25th	50th	75th	90th	95th	5th	10th	25th	50th	75th	90th	95th
1	90th	97	97	98	100	101	102	103	52	53	53	54	55	55	56
	95th	100	101	102	104	105	106	107	56	57	57	58	59	59	60
2	90th	98	99	100	101	103	104	105	57	58	58	59	60	61	61
	95th	102	103	104	105	107	108	109	61	62	62	63	64	65	65
3	90th	100	100	102	103	104	106	106	61	62	62	63	64	64	65
	95th	104	104	105	107	108	109	110	65	66	66	67	68	68	69
4	90th	101	102	103	104	106	107	108	64	64	65	66	67	67	68
	95th	105	106	107	108	110	111	112	68	68	69	70	71	71	72
5	90th	103	103	105	106	107	109	109	66	67	67	68	69	69	70
	95th	107	107	108	110	111	112	113	70	71	71	72	73	73	74
6	90th	104	105	106	108	109	110	111	68	68	69	70	70	71	72
	95th	108	109	110	111	113	114	115	72	72	73	74	74	75	76
7	90th	106	107	108	109	111	112	113	69	70	70	71	72	72	73
	95th	110	111	112	113	115	116	116	73	74	74	75	76	76	77
8	90th	108	109	110	111	113	114	114	71	71	71	72	73	74	74
	95th	112	112	114	115	116	118	118	75	75	75	76	77	78	78

Continued

From The Fourth Report on the Diagnosis, Evaluation, and Treatment of High Blood Pressure in Children and Adolescents, 2004.
*Blood pressure percentile was determined by a single measurement.
†Height percentile was determined by standard growth curves.

Blood Pressure Levels for the 90th and 95th Percentiles of Blood Pressure for Girls Age 1 to 17 Years by Percentiles of Height—cont'd

Age, Years	Blood Pressure Percentile*	Systolic Blood Pressure by Percentile of Height, mm Hg†							Diastolic Blood Pressure by Percentile of Height, mm Hg†						
		5th	10th	25th	50th	75th	90th	95th	5th	10th	25th	50th	75th	90th	95th
9	90th	110	110	112	113	114	116	116	72	72	72	73	74	75	75
	95th	114	114	115	117	118	119	120	76	76	76	77	78	79	79
10	90th	112	112	114	115	116	118	118	73	73	73	74	75	76	76
	95th	116	116	117	119	120	121	122	77	77	77	78	79	80	80
11	90th	114	114	116	117	118	119	120	74	74	74	75	76	77	77
	95th	118	118	119	121	122	123	124	78	78	78	79	80	81	81
12	90th	116	116	117	119	120	121	122	75	75	75	76	77	78	78
	95th	119	120	121	123	124	125	126	79	79	79	80	81	82	82
13	90th	117	118	119	121	122	123	124	76	76	76	77	78	79	79
	95th	121	122	123	124	126	127	128	80	80	80	81	82	83	83
14	90th	119	120	121	122	124	125	125	77	77	77	78	79	80	80
	95th	123	123	125	126	127	129	129	81	81	81	82	83	84	84
15	90th	120	121	122	123	125	126	127	78	78	78	79	80	81	81
	95th	124	125	126	127	129	130	131	82	82	82	83	84	85	85
16	90th	121	122	123	124	126	127	128	78	78	79	80	81	81	82
	95th	125	126	127	128	130	131	132	82	82	83	84	85	85	86
17	90th	122	122	123	125	126	127	128	78	79	79	80	81	81	82
	95th	125	126	127	129	130	131	132	82	83	83	84	85	85	86

From The Fourth Report on the Diagnosis, Evaluation, and Treatment of High Blood Pressure in Children and Adolescents, 2004.
*Blood pressure percentile was determined by a single measurement.
†Height percentile was determined by standard growth curves.

CHAPTER 12

BREASTS AND AXILLAE

EQUIPMENT

- ▦ Ruler (if mass detected)
- ▦ Flashlight with transilluminator (if mass detected)
- ▦ Glass slide and cytologic fixative (for nipple discharge)
- ▦ Small pillow or folded towel

EXAMINATION

TECHNIQUE   **FINDINGS**

FEMALES

With patient seated and arms hanging loosely, inspect both breasts

Inspect all quadrants and tail of Spence as shown in figure. If necessary, lift breasts with fingertips to expose lower and lateral aspects.

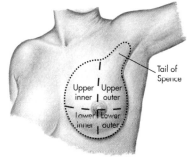

Tail of Spence

Upper inner | Upper outer

Lower inner | Lower outer

▦ *Size/shape/symmetry*

▦ *Texture/contour*

EXPECTED: Convex, pendulous, or conical. Frequently asymmetric in size.

EXPECTED: Smooth and uninterrupted.

TECHNIQUE	**FINDINGS**
	UNEXPECTED: Dimpling or peau d'orange appearance. Changes or asymmetric appearance.
■ *Skin color*	**EXPECTED:** Consistent color **UNEXPECTED:** Areas of discoloration or asymmetric appearance.
■ *Venous patterns*	**EXPECTED:** Bilateral venous networks, although pronounced generally only in pregnant or obese women. **UNEXPECTED:** Unilateral network.
■ *Markings*	**EXPECTED:** Long-standing nevi. Supernumerary nipples possible (but could be a clue to other congenital abnormalities). **UNEXPECTED:** Changing or tender nevi. Lesions.

Inspect areolae and nipples

■ *Size/shape/symmetry*	**EXPECTED:** Areolae round or oval, bilaterally equal or nearly equal. Nipples bilaterally equal or nearly equal in size and usually everted, although one or both sometimes inverted. **UNEXPECTED:** Recent unilateral nipple inversion or retraction.
■ *Color*	**EXPECTED:** Areolae and nipples pink to brown. **UNEXPECTED:** Nonhomogeneous in color.
■ *Texture/contour*	**EXPECTED:** Areolae smooth, except for Montgomery tubercles. Nipples smooth or wrinkled. **UNEXPECTED:** Areolae with suppurative or tender Montgomery tubercles or with peau d'orange appearance.

TECHNIQUE	**FINDINGS**

Nipples crusting, cracking, or with discharge.

With patient in the following positions, reinspect both breasts

- *Arms extended over head, or flexed behind the neck*

EXPECTED, ALL POSITIONS: Breasts bilaterally symmetric with even contour.

- *Hands pressed on hips with shoulders rolled forward or pushed together in front*
- *Seated and leaning over*
- *Recumbent*

UNEXPECTED: Dimpling, retraction, deviation, or fixation of breasts.

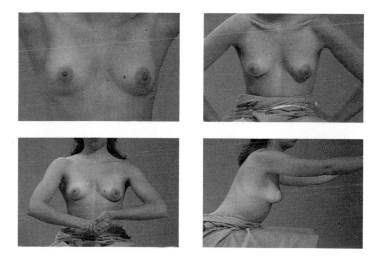

With patient seated and arms hanging loosely, palpate breasts

Chest wall sweep. Place the palm of your right hand at the patient's right clavicle at the sternum. Sweep downward from the clavicle to the nipple feeling for superficial lumps. Repeat the sweep until you have covered the

EXPECTED: Tissue smooth, free of lumps.
UNEXPECTED: Lumps or nodules. Reassess with additional palpation and characterize any masses by location, size, shape, consistency, tenderness,

TECHNIQUE	**FINDINGS**

entire right chest wall. Repeat the procedure using your left hand for the left chest wall.

mobility, delineation of borders, retraction. Use transillumination to assess presence of fluid in masses.

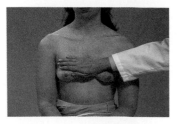

Bimanual digital palpation. Place one hand, palmar surface facing up, under the patient's right breast. Position your hand so that it acts as a flat surface against which to compress the breast tissue. Walk the fingers of the other hand across the breast tissue, feeling for lumps as you compress the tissue between your fingers and your flat hand. Repeat the procedure for the other breast.

EXPECTED: Tissue generally firm, nontender, free of lumps. During menstrual cycle, cyclic pattern of breast enlargement, increased nodularity, tenderness.

UNEXPECTED: Lumps or nodules. Reassess with additional palpation and characterize any masses by location, size, shape, consistency, tenderness, mobility, delineation of borders, retraction. Use transillumination to assess presence of fluid in masses.

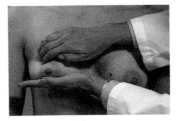

With patient seated, palpate for lymph nodes

Right axilla: Support patient's lower right arm with your right hand while examining right axilla with your left hand. With palmar surface of fingers, reach deep into

UNEXPECTED: Nodes, especially in supraclavicular area. Describe nodes by location, size, shape, consistency, tenderness,

TECHNIQUE	**FINDINGS**

hollow, pushing firmly upward; then bring fingers down, gently rolling soft tissue against chest wall and axilla. Explore apex, medial, lateral aspects along rib cage; lateral aspects along upper surface of arm; and anterior and posterior walls of axilla. Repeat mirror image of this maneuver for left axilla.

Supraclavicular area: Hook fingers over clavicle and rotate over supraclavicular fossa while patient turns head toward same side and raises shoulder. Infraclavicular area: Palpate along the clavicle using a rotary motion with your fingers.

fixation, delineation of borders.

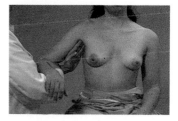

With patient supine, continue palpation of breast tissue

Have patient put one hand behind head. Place a towel under shoulder of same side, as shown in figure on p. 136. Compress breast tissue between fingers and chest wall, using rotary motion of fingers. Using finger pads, systematically palpate each breast in all four quadrants, including tail of Spence and over areolae. Push gently but firmly toward chest while rotating fingers clockwise or counterclockwise, following a vertical strip, concentric circle, or wedge pattern. At each point press inward, using three depths of palpation: light, medium, and deep.

Return to the nipple and with two fingers gently depress the tissue inward into the well behind the areola. Repeat palpation maneuvers for other breast.

EXPECTED: Tissue generally dense, firm, elastic but sometimes lobular. May be fine and granular in older women. Inframammary ridge may be felt along lower edge of breast. During menstrual cycle, cyclic pattern of breast enlargement, increased nodularity, tenderness.

UNEXPECTED: Lumps or nodules. Characterize any masses by location, size, shape, consistency, tenderness, mobility, delineation of

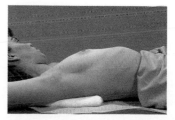

TECHNIQUE	**FINDINGS**
	borders, retraction. Use transillumination to assess presence of fluid in masses. **EXPECTED:** Fingers and tissue move easily inward. **UNEXPECTED:** Lump, mass; absence of well behind areola.

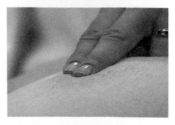

MALES

Inspect both breasts
- *Size/shape/symmetry*
- *Surface characteristics*

EXPECTED: Even with chest wall. Sometimes convex (especially in overweight men).
UNEXPECTED: Enlarged breasts.

Inspect areolae and nipples
- *Size/shape/symmetry*

EXPECTED: Areolae round or oval, bilaterally equal or nearly equal. Nipples bilaterally equal or nearly equal in size and usually everted, although one or both sometimes inverted.
UNEXPECTED: Recent unilateral nipple inversion or retraction.

- *Color*

EXPECTED: Areolae and nipples pink to brown.
UNEXPECTED: Nonhomogeneous in color.

- *Texture/contour*

EXPECTED: Areolae smooth, except for Montgomery tubercles. Nipples smooth or wrinkled.

TECHNIQUE	FINDINGS
	UNEXPECTED: Areolae with suppurative or tender Montgomery tubercles or with peau d'orange appearance. Nipples crusting, cracking, or with discharge.

Palpate breasts and over areolae

■ *Palpate briefly, following palpation steps for females.*	**EXPECTED:** Thin layer of fatty tissue overlying muscle. Thick layer in obese men may give appearance of breast enlargement. Firm disk of glandular tissue sometimes evident. **UNEXPECTED:** Lumps or nodules,

With patient seated and arms flexed at elbows, palpate for lymph nodes

Palpate as described for females.	**UNEXPECTED:** Nodes, especially in supraclavicular area. Describe nodes by location, size, shape, consistency, tenderness, fixation, delineation of borders.

AIDS TO DIFFERENTIAL DIAGNOSIS

ABNORMALITY	DESCRIPTION
Fibrocystic changes	See table of differentiating signs and symptoms, p. 138.
Fibroadenoma	
Malignant breast tumors	
Adult gynecomastia	Smooth, firm, mobile, tender disk of breast tissue behind areola in males, unilaterally or bilaterally.
Mastitis	Swelling, tenderness, heat; patient may have fever. Abscess—pus-filled, hardened mass that is fluctuant, hard, erythematous.

Differentiating Signs and Symptoms of Breast Masses

	Fibrocystic Changes	Fibroadenoma	Cancer
Age, years	20-49	15-55	30-80
Occurrence	Usually bilateral	Usually bilateral	Usually unilateral
Number	Multiple or single	Single; may be multiple	Single
Shape	Round	Round or discoid	Irregular or stellate
Consistency	Soft to firm; tense	Firm, rubbery	Hard, stonelike
Mobility	Mobile	Mobile	Fixed
Retraction signs	Absent	Absent	Often present
Tenderness	Usually tender	Usually nontender	Usually nontender
Delimitation	Well delineated	Well delineated	Poorly delineated; irregular
Variation with menses	Yes	No	No

PEDIATRIC VARIATIONS

EXAMINATION

Palpate and compress nipples

EXPECTED: Breast enlargement is not unusual in newborns. "Witch's milk" may be expressed.

Assess stage of pubertal development

In females, assess the stage of breast development.

EXPECTED: The duration and tempo of each stage and sequence are quite variable between individuals. Tanner stages of breast development:

TECHNIQUE	FINDINGS

M_1 —Tanner 1 (preadolescent). Only the nipple is raised above the level of the breast, as in the child.

M_2 —Tanner 2. Budding stage; bud-shaped elevation of the areola; areola increased in diameter and surrounding area slightly elevated.

M_3 —Tanner 3. Breast and areola enlarged. No contour separation.

M_4 —Tanner 4. Increasing fat deposits. The areola forms a secondary elevation above that of the breast. This secondary mound occurs in approximately half of all girls and in some cases persists in adulthood.

M_5 —Tanner 5 (adult stage). The areola is (usually) part of general breast contour and is strongly pigmented. Nipple projects.

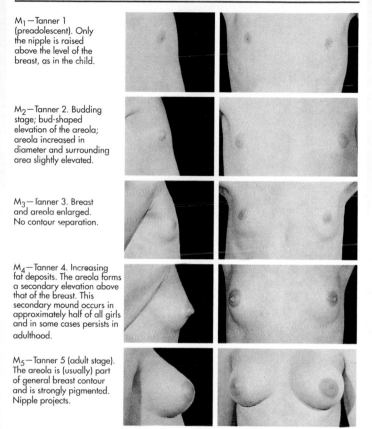

Five stages of breast development in females. *From Van Wieringen et al, 1971. Reprinted by permission of Kluwer Academic Publishers.*

AIDS TO DIFFERENTIAL DIAGNOSIS

ABNORMALITY	DESCRIPTION
Gynecomastia	Enlargement of breast tissue in boys caused by puberty, hormonal imbalance, testicular or pituitary tumors, or medications containing estrogens or steroids. Thorough investigation should be conducted to rule out pathologic conditions.

SAMPLE DOCUMENTATION

Subjective. A 42-year-old female noticed a "knot" in her right lower breast last week. Denies nipple discharge or skin changes. Reports normal mammogram 2 years ago. Has never had a breast lump before. Currently on last day of menses. Has breast tenderness just before menses but denies breast pain today. No family history of breast cancer.
Objective. Breasts moderate size, conical shape, left slightly larger than right. No skin lesions, contour smooth without dimpling or retraction; venous pattern symmetric. Nipple symmetric, without discharge; Montgomery tubercles bilaterally. Tissue dense, particularly in upper quadrants; 3 × 2 cm soft mass in lower left quadrant of right breast. Mobile, nontender. No nipple discharge expressed. No supraclavicular, infraclavicular, or axillary lymphadenopathy.

CHAPTER 13

ABDOMEN

EQUIPMENT

- Stethoscope
- Skin-marking pencil
- Centimeter ruler or tape measure
- Reflex hammer or tongue blade

EXAMINATION

Have patient in the supine position to start the examination. Approach the patient from the right side.

TECHNIQUE	FINDINGS
Inspect abdomen in all four quadrants (see box on p. 142)	
■ *Skin color/characteristics*	**EXPECTED:** Usual color variations, such as paleness or tanning lines. Fine venous network (venous return toward head above umbilicus, toward feet below umbilicus).
	UNEXPECTED: Generalized color changes, such as jaundice or cyanosis. Glistening taut appearance. Bluish periumbilical discoloration, bruises, other localized discoloration. Striae, lesions or nodules, a pearl-like enlarged umbilical node, scars.
■ *Contour/symmetry* Begin seated to patient's right to enhance shadows and	**EXPECTED:** Flat, rounded, or scaphoid. Contralateral areas symmetric. Maximum height of

TECHNIQUE	FINDINGS
contouring. Inspect while patient breathes comfortably and while patient holds a deep breath. Assess symmetry, first seated at patient's side, then standing behind patient's head.	convexity at umbilicus. Abdomen remains smooth and symmetric while patient holds breath. **UNEXPECTED:** Umbilicus displaced upward, downward, or laterally or is inflamed, swollen, or bulging. Any distention (symmetric or asymmetric), bulges, or masses while breathing comfortably or holding breath.
■ *Surface motion*	**EXPECTED:** Smooth, even motion with respiration. Females mostly costal; males mostly abdominal. Pulsation in upper midline in thin aduls. **UNEXPECTED:** Limited motion with respiration in adult

Anatomic Correlates of the Four Quadrants of the Abdomen

Right Upper Quadrant
Liver and gallbladder
Pylorus
Duodenum
Head of pancreas
Right adrenal gland
Portion of right kidney
Hepatic flexure of colon
Portions of ascending and
  transverse colon

Left Upper Quadrant
Left lobe of liver
Spleen
Stomach
Body of pancreas
Left adrenal gland
Portion of left kidney
Splenic flexure of colon
Portions of transverse and
  descending colon

Right Lower Quadrant
Lower pole of right kidney
Cecum and appendix
Portion of ascending colon
Bladder (if distended)
Ovary and salpinx
Uterus (if enlarged)
Right spermatic cord
Right ureter

Left Lower Quadrant
Lower pole of left kidney
Sigmoid colon
Portion of descending colon
Bladder (if distended)
Ovary and salpinx
Uterus (if enlarged)
Left spermatic cord
Left ureter

TECHNIQUE   **FINDINGS**

males. Rippling movement
(peristalsis) or marked pulsation.

Inspect abdominal muscles as patient raises head

EXPECTED: No masses or
protrusions.
UNEXPECTED: Masses,
protrusion of the umbilicus and
other hernia signs, or muscle
separation.

Auscultate with stethoscope diaphragm

■ *Frequency and character of
bowel sounds*
Warm stethoscope diaphragm,
and hold with light pressure.
May auscultate at a single site,
but auscultate in all quadrants
if you have reason to be
concerned.

EXPECTED: Five to 35
irregular clicks and gurgles per
minute. Borborygmi or
increased sounds due to hunger.
UNEXPECTED: Increased
sounds unrelated to hunger,
high-pitched tinkling, or
decreased or absent sounds
after 5 minutes of listening.

■ *Liver and spleen*

EXPECTED: Silent.
UNEXPECTED: Friction rubs.

Auscultate with stethoscope bell

■ *Vascular sounds*
Listen with stethoscope bell in
epigastric region, over aorta,
and over renal, iliac, and
femoral arteries.

EXPECTED: No bruits,
venous hum, or friction rubs.
UNEXPECTED: Bruits in
aortic, renal, iliac, or femoral
arteries.

Percussion Notes of the Abdomen

Note	Description	Location
Tympany	Musical note of higher pitch than resonance	Over air-filled viscera
Hyperresonance	Pitch lies between tympany and resonance	Base of left lung
Resonance	Sustained note of moderate pitch	Over lung tissue and sometimes over abdomen
Dullness	Short, high-pitched note with little resonance	Over solid organs adjacent to air-filled structures

Modified from AH Robins Co.

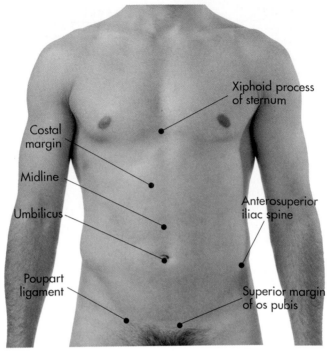

Xiphoid process
of sternum

Costal
margin

Midline

Umbilicus

Anterosuperior
iliac spine

Poupart
ligament

Superior margin
of os pubis

From Thompson and Wilson, 1996.

TECHNIQUE	FINDINGS
◼ *Epigastric region and around umbilicus*	**EXPECTED:** No venous hum. **UNEXPECTED:** Venous hum.

Percuss abdomen

NOTE: Percussion can be done independently or concurrently with palpation.

◼ *Tone*
Percuss in all quadrants.

EXPECTED: Tympany predominant. Dullness over organs and solid masses. Dullness in suprapubic area from distended bladder. See table on p. 143 for percussion notes.
UNEXPECTED: Dullness predominant.

◼ *Liver span*
To determine lower liver

EXPECTED: Lower border usually begins at or slightly

TECHNIQUE

FINDINGS

border, percuss upward at right midclavicular line, as shown in figure below, and mark with a pen where tympany changes to dullness. To determine upper liver border, percuss downward at right midclavicular line from an area of resonance, and mark change to dullness. Measure the distance between marks to estimate vertical span.

- *Spleen*
Percuss just posterior to midaxillary line on left, beginning at areas of lung

below costal margin. Upper border usually begins at fifth to seventh intercostal space Span generally ranges from 6 to 12 cm in adults.

UNEXPECTED: Lower liver border more than 2 to 3 cm below costal margin. Upper liver border below seventh or above fifth intercostal span. Span greater than 12 cm or less than 6 cm.

EXPECTED: Small area of dullness from sixth to tenth rib. Tympany before and after deep breath.

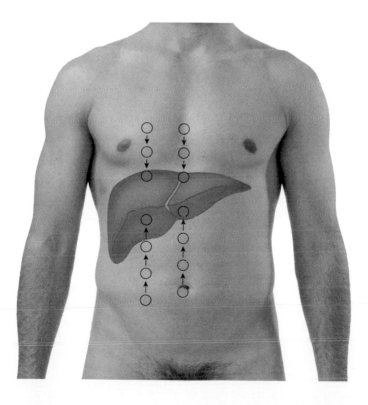

TECHNIQUE	FINDINGS

resonance and moving in several directions. Percuss lowest intercostal space in left anterior axillary line before and after patient takes deep breath.

■ *Stomach*

UNEXPECTED: Large area of dullness (check for full stomach or feces-filled intestine). Tone change from tympany to dullness with inspiration.

Percuss in area of left lower anterior rib cage and left epigastric region.

EXPECTED: Tympany of gastric air bubble (lower than intestine tympany).
UNEXPECTED: Dullnes.

Lightly palpate abdomen

Stand at patient's side (usually right). Systematically palpate all quadrants, avoiding areas previously identified as trouble spots. With palmar surfaces of fingers, depress abdominal wall up to 1 cm with light, even motion. Identify areas of peritoneal irritation by assessing for cutaneous hypersensitivity.

EXPECTED: Abdomen smooth with consistent softness. Possible tension from palpating too deeply, cold hands, or ticklishness.
UNEXPECTED: Muscular tension or resistance, tenderness, or masses. If resistance is present, place pillow under patient's knees, and ask patient to breathe slowly through mouth. Feel for relaxation of rectus abdominis muscles on expiration. Continuing tension signals involuntary response to abdominal rigidity. Cutaneous hypersensitivity.

Palpate abdomen with moderate pressure

Using same hand position as above, palpate all quadrants again, this time with moderate pressure.

EXPECTED: Soft, nontender
UNEXPECTED: Tenderness.

TECHNIQUE	FINDINGS

Deeply palpate abdomen

With same hand position as above, repeat palpation in all quadrants, pressing deeply and evenly into abdominal wall. Move fingers back and forth over abdominal contents. Use bimanual technique—exerting pressure with top hand and concentrating on sensation with bottom hand, as shown in figure at right—if obesity or muscular resistance makes deep palpation difficult. To help determine whether masses are superficial or intraabdominal, have patient lift head from examining table to contract abdominal muscles and obscure intraabdominal masses.

EXPECTED: Possible sensation of abdominal wall sliding back and forth. Possible awareness of borders of rectus abdominis muscles, aorta, and portions of colon. Possible tenderness over cecum, sigmoid colon, and aorta and in midline near xiphoid process.

UNEXPECTED: Bulges, masses, tenderness unrelated to deep palpation of cecum, sigmoid colon, aorta, xiphoid process. Note location, size, shape, consistency, tenderness, pulsation, mobility, movement (with respiration) of any masses.

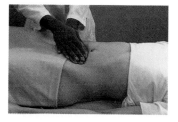

■ *Umbilical ring and umbilicus*
Palpate umbilical ring and around umbilicus. Note whether ring is incomplete or soft in center.

EXPECTED: Umbilical ring circular and free of irregularities. Umbilicus either slightly inverted or everted.

UNEXPECTED: Bulges, nodules, granulation. Protruding umbilicus.

■ *Liver*
Place left hand under patient at eleventh and twelfth ribs, lifting to elevate liver toward abdominal wall. Place right hand on abdomen, fingers extended toward head with

EXPECTED: Usually liver is not palpable. If felt, liver edge should be firm, smooth, even.

UNEXPECTED: Tenderness, nodules, or irregularity.

TECHNIQUE   **FINDINGS**

tips on right midclavicular
line below level of liver dullness,
as shown in figure at right.
Alternatively, place right hand
parallel to right costal margin,
as shown in figure at right,
below. Press right hand gently
but deeply in and up. Ask
patient to breathe comfortably
a few times and then take a
deep breath. Feel for liver edge
as diaphragm pushes it down.
If palpable, repeat maneuver
medially and laterally to costal
margin.

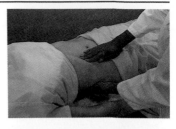

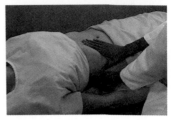

■ *Gallbladder*
Palpate below liver margin at
lateral border of rectus
abdominis muscle.

EXPECTED: Gallbladder not
palpable.
UNEXPECTED: Palpable,
tender or nontender. If tender
(possible cholecystitis), palpate
deeply during inspiration and
observe for pain (Murphy sign).

■ *Spleen*
Reach across patient with left
hand, place it beneath patient
over left costovertebral angle,
and lift spleen anteriorly toward
abdominal wall. As shown in
figure, place right hand on
abdomen below left costal
margin and—using findings
from percussion—gently press
fingertips inward toward
spleen while asking patient to
take a deep breath. Feel for
spleen as it moves downward
toward fingers.
Repeat with patient lying on
right side, as shown in figure
below, with hips and knees
flexed. Press inward with left

EXPECTED: Spleen usually
not palpable by either method.
UNEXPECTED: Palpable
spleen.

TECHNIQUE	FINDINGS

hand while using fingertips
of right hand to feel edge
of spleen.

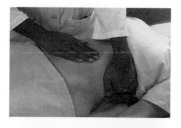

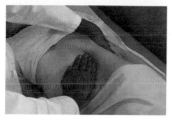

- *Left kidney*
Standing on patient's right,
reach across with left hand,
and place over left flank;
then place right hand at
patient's left costal margin.
Ask patient to inhale deeply,
while you elevate left flank
and palpate deeply with right
hand.

EXPECTED: Left kidney
usually not palpable.
UNEXPECTED: Pain.

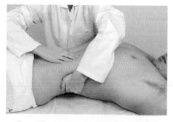

From Thompson and Wilson, 1996.

TECHNIQUE	**FINDINGS**
■ *Right kidney* Standing on patient's right, place left hand under right flank, then place right hand at patient's right costal margin. Ask patient to inhale deeply while you elevate right flank and palpate deeply with right hand.	**EXPECTED:** If palpable, right kidney should be smooth and firm with rounded edges. **UNEXPECTED:** Tenderness.

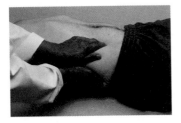

■ *Aorta* Palpate deeply slightly to left of midline, and feel for aortic pulsation. As an alternative technique, place palmar surface of hands with fingers extended on midline; press fingers deeply inward on each side of aorta, and feel for pulsation. For thin patients, use one hand, placing thumb and fingers on either side of aorta.	**EXPECTED:** Pulsation anterior in direction. **UNEXPECTED:** Prominent lateral pulsation.

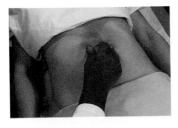

■ *Urinary bladder* Percuss distended bladder to help determine outline, then palpate.	**EXPECTED:** Ordinarily not palpable unless distended with urine. If distended, bladder should be smooth, round, and

TECHNIQUE	**FINDINGS**

| | tense and on percussion will elicit lower note than surrounding air-filled intestines. **UNEXPECTED:** Palpable when not distended with urine. |

Elicit abdominal reflexes

| Stroke each quadrant of abdomen with end of reflex hammer or tongue blade edge. Elicit upper abdominal reflexes by stroking upward and away from umbilicus; elicit lower abdominal reflexes by stroking downward and away from umbilicus. | **EXPECTED:** With each stroke, contraction of rectus abdominis muscles and pulling of umbilicus toward stroked side. Reflex may be diminished in patient who is obese or whose abdominal muscles were stretched during pregnancy. **UNEXPECTED:** Absence of reflex. |

With patient sitting, percuss costovertebral angles

| Stand behind patient. *Right side:* Place left hand over right costovertebral angle and strike with ulnar surface of right fist. *Left side:* Repeat with hands reversed. | **EXPECTED:** No tenderness. **UNEXPECTED:** Kidney tenderness or pain. |

Pain assessment

| Keep eyes on patient's face while examining abdomen. To help characterize pain, have patient cough, take a deep breath, jump, or walk. Ask whether patient is hungry. | **UNEXPECTED:** Unwillingness to move, nausea, vomiting, areas of localized tenderness. Lack of hunger. See box and table on p. 152. |

Some Causes of Pain Perceived in Anatomic Regions

Right Upper Quadrant
- Duodenal ulcer
- Hepatitis
- Hepatomegaly
- Pneumonia

Right Lower Quadrant
- Appendicitis
- Salpingitis
- Ovarian cyst
- Ruptured ectopic pregnancy
- Renal/ureteral stone
- Strangulated hernia
- Meckel diverticulitis
- Regional ileitis
- Perforated cecum

Periumbilical
- Intestinal obstruction
- Acute pancreatitis
- Early appendicitis
- Mesenteric thrombosis
- Aortic aneurysm
- Diverticulitis

Modified from Judge et al., 1988.

Left Upper Quadrant
- Ruptured spleen
- Gastric ulcer
- Aortic aneurysm
- Perforated colon
- Pneumonia

Left Lower Quadrant
- Sigmoid diverticulitis
- Salpingitis
- Ovarian cyst
- Ruptured ectopic pregnancy
- Renal/ureteral stone
- Strangulated hernia
- Perforated colon
- Regional ileitis
- Ulcerative colitis

Quality and Onset of Abdominal Pain

Characteristic	Possible Related Condition
Burning	Peptic ulcer
Cramping	Biliary colic, gastroenteritis
Colic	Appendicitis with impacted feces; renal stone
Aching	Appendiceal irritation
Knifelike	Pancreatitis
Gradual onset	Infection
Sudden onset	Duodenal ulcer, acute pancreatitis, obstruction, perforation

Iliopsoas muscle test

Use test for suspected appendicitis. With patient supine, place hand over lower thigh. Ask patient to

UNEXPECTED: Lower quadrant pain.

TECHNIQUE	FINDINGS

raise leg, flexing at hip, while
you push downward.

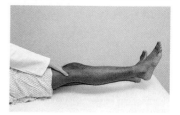

Obturator muscle test

Use test for suspected ruptured
appendix or pelvic abscess.
With patient supine, ask patient
to flex right leg at hip and bend
knee to 90 degrees. Hold leg
just above knee, grasp ankle,
and rotate leg laterally and
medially, as shown in figure
at right.

UNEXPECTED: Pain in
hypogastric region.

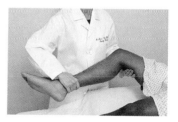

AIDS TO DIFFERENTIAL DIAGNOSIS

ABNORMALITY	DESCRIPTION
Hiatal hernia with esophagitis	Epigastric pain and/or heartburn that worsens with reclining and is relieved by sitting or with antacids; water brash; or dysphagia. Sudden onset of vomiting, pain, complete dysphagia are symptoms of hernia incarceration.
Gastroesophageal reflux disease (GERD)	Backward flow of acid from stomach up into esophagus. Patients may experience heartburn, a sour taste of acid in the back of the throat, or hoarseness. Symptoms in infants and children include regurgitation and vomiting. Condition can cause respiratory

ABNORMALITY	DESCRIPTION
	problems from aspiration and bleeding from esophagitis.
Duodenal ulcer	Localized epigastric pain occurring with empty stomach that is relieved with food or antacids. Tenderness on palpation of abdomen for anterior-wall ulcers. Hematemesis, melena, dizziness or syncope, decreased blood pressure, increased pulse rate, decreased hematocrit level are symptoms of upper gastrointestinal (GI) bleeding. Signs of an acute abdomen could indicate perforation of duodenum, **a life-threatening event.**
Acute diarrhea	Abrupt onset, lasts less than 2 weeks. Common symptoms include abdominal pain, diarrhea, nausea, vomiting, fever, and tenesmus. Caused by viral, bacterial or parasitic infection. Consider food poisoning if diarrhea develops in two or more persons following ingestion of the same food.
Crohn disease	Cramping diarrhea, mild bleeding, occurs anywhere in GI tract; fissure, fistula abscess formation; periumbilical colic; malabsorption; folate deficiency.
Ulcerative colitis	Mild to severe symptoms; bloody, watery diarrhea; no localized peritoneal signs; weight loss, fatigue, general debility.
Irritable bowel syndrome (IBS)	Functional disorder of the intestine that produces a cluster of symptoms, usually abdominal pain, bloating, constipation, diarrhea. Some patients with IBS experience alternating diarrhea

ABNORMALITY	DESCRIPTION
	and constipation. Mucus may be present around or within the stool.
Colon cancer	Occult blood in stool. History of changes in frequency or character of stool. Lesion may be felt on rectal examination. Tumor may be palpated in right or left lower quadrant.
Hepatitis	Jaundice, anorexia, abdominal gastric discomfort, clay-colored stools, tea-colored urine. Enlarged liver. Caused by viral infection, alcohol, drugs, or toxins.
Cirrhosis	Ascites, jaundice, prominent abdominal vasculature, cutaneous spider angiomas, dark urine, light-colored stools, spleen enlargement. Complaints of fatigue. Muscle wasting in late stages.
Cholecystitis	*Acute:* Pain in upper right quadrant with radiation around midtorso to right scapular region. Pain abrupt and severe, lasting 2 to 4 hours. *Chronic:* Repeated acute attacks; a scarred and contracted gallbladder; fat intolerance, flatulence, nausea, anorexia, nonspecific abdominal pain, and tenderness of right hypochondriac region.
Chronic pancreatitis	Unremitting abdominal pain, epigastric tenderness, weight loss, steatorrhea, glucose intolerance.
Pyelonephritis	Flank pain, bacteriuria, pyuria, dysuria, nocturia, urinary frequency. Possible costovertebral angle tenderness.
Renal calculi	Fever, hematuria, flank pain that may extend to groin and genitals.

ABNORMALITY	DESCRIPTION
Appendicitis	Initially, periumbilical or epigastric pain; colicky; later becomes localized to right lower quadrant, often at McBurney point.

Abdominal Signs Associated with Common Abnormalities

Sign	Description	Associated Conditions
Aaron	Pain or distress occurs in the area of patient's heart or stomach on palpation of McBurney point	Appendicitis
Ballance	Fixed dullness to percussion in left flank and dullness in right flank that disappear on change of position	Peritoneal irritation
Blumberg	Rebound tenderness	Peritoneal irritation, appendicitis
Cullen	Ecchymosis around umbilicus	Hemoperitoneum, pancreatitis, ectopic pregnancy
Dance	Absence of bowel sounds in right lower quadrant	Intussusception
Grey Turner	Ecchymosis of flanks	Hemoperitoneum, pancreatitis
Kehr	Abdominal pain radiating to left shoulder	Spleen rupture, renal calculi, ectopic pregnancy
Markle (heel jar)	Patient stands with straightened knees, then raises up on toes, relaxes, and allows heels to hit floor, thus jarring body; action will cause abdominal pain if positive	Peritoneal irritation, appendicitis

Abdominal Signs Associated with Common Abnormalities—cont'd

Sign	Description	Associated Conditions
McBurney	Rebound tenderness and sharp pain when McBurney point is palpated	Appendicitis
Murphy	Abrupt cessation of inspiration on palpation of gallbladder	Cholecystitis
Romberg-Howship	Pain down medial aspect of thigh to knees	Strangulated obturator hernia
Rovsing	Right lower quadrant pain intensified by left lower quadrant abdominal palpation palpation	Peritoneal irritation, appendicitis

Differential Diagnosis: Common Conditions Producing Acute Abdominal Pain

Condition	Usual Pain Characteristics	Possible Associated Findings
Appendicitis	Initially periumbilical or epigastric; colicky; later becomes localized to RLQ, often at McBurney point	Guarding, tenderness; + iliopsoas and + obturator signs; RLQ skin hyperesthesia; anorexia, nausea, or vomiting after onset of pain; low-grade fever; + Aaron, Rovsing, Markle, and McBurney signs*
Peritonitis	Onset sudden or gradual; pain generalized or localized, dull or severe and unrelenting; guarding; pain on deep inspiration	Shallow respiration; + Blumberg, Markle, and Ballance signs; reduced bowel sounds, nausea and vomiting; + obturator and iliopsoas tests
Cholecystitis	Severe, unrelenting RUQ or epigastric pain; may be referred to right subscapular area	RUQ tenderness and rigidity, + Murphy sign, palpable gallbladder, anorexia, vomiting, fever, possible jaundice
Pancreatitis	Dramatic, sudden, excruciating LUQ, epigastric, or umbilical pain; may be present in one or both flanks; may be referred to left shoulder	Epigastric tenderness, vomiting, fever; shock; + Grey Turner sign; + Cullen sign; both signs occur 2-3 days after onset
Salpingitis	Lower quadrant, worse on left	Nausea, vomiting, fever, suprapubic tenderness, rigid abdomen, pain on pelvic examination
Pelvic inflammatory disease	Lower quadrant, increases with activity	Tender adnexa and cervix, cervical discharge, dyspareunia
Diverticulitis	Epigastric, radiating down left side of abdomen especially after eating; may be referred to back	Flatulence, borborygmus, diarrhea, dysuria, tenderness on palpation
Perforated gastric or duodenal ulcer	Abrupt RUQ; may be referred to shoulders	Abdominal free air and distention with increased resonance over liver; tenderness in epigastrium or RUQ; rigid abdominal wall, rebound tenderness

Intestinal obstruction	Abrupt, severe, spasmodic; referred to epigastrium, umbilicus	Distention, minimal rebound tenderness, vomiting, localized tenderness, visible peristalsis; bowel sounds absent (with paralytic obstruction) or hyperactive high-pitched (with mechanical obstruction)
Volvulus	Referred to hypogastrium and umbilicus	Distention, nausea, vomiting, guarding; sigmoid loop volvulus may be palpable
Leaking abdominal aneurysm	Steady throbbing midline over aneurysm; may radiate to back, flank	Nausea, vomiting, abdominal mass, bruit
Biliary stones, colic	Episodic, severe, RUQ, or epigastrium lasting 15 min to several hours; may be referred to subscapular area, especially right	RUQ tenderness, soft abdominal wall, anorexia, vomiting, jaundice, subnormal temperature
Renal calculi	Intense; flank, extending to groin and genitals; may be episodic	Fever, hematuria; + Kehr sign
Ectopic pregnancy	Lower quadrant; referred to shoulder; with rupture is agonizing	Hypogastric tenderness, symptoms of pregnancy, spotting, irregular menses, soft abdominal wall, mass on bimanual pelvic examination; ruptured: shock, rigid abdominal wall, distention; + Kehr, Cullen signs
Ruptured ovarian cyst	Lower quadrant, steady, increases with cough or motion	Vomiting, low-grade fever, anorexia, tenderness on pelvic examination
Splenic rupture	Intense; LUQ, radiating to left shoulder; may worsen with foot of bed elevated	Shock, pallor, lowered temperature

See Table 13-3 for explanation of signs.
LUQ, left upper quadrant; RLQ, right lower quadrant; RUQ, right upper quadrant.

Differential Diagnosis: Common Conditions Producing Chronic Abdominal Pain

Condition	Usual Pain Characteristics	Possible Associated Findings
Irritable bowel syndrome	Hypogastric pain; crampy, variable, infrequent; associated with bowel function	Negative physical examination. Pain associated with gas, bloating, distention; relief with passage of flatus, feces
Lactose intolerance	Crampy pain after eating milk or milk products	Associated diarrhea; negative physical examination
Diverticular disease	Localized pain	Abdominal tenderness, fever
Constipation	Colicky or dull and steady pain that does not progress or worsen	Fecal mass palpable, stool in rectum
Uterine fibroids	Pain related to menses, intercourse	Palpable myoma(s)
Hernia	Localized pain that increases with exertion or lifting	Hernia on physical examination
Esophagitis/GERD	Burning, gnawing pain in midepigastrium, worsens with recumbency	Negative physical examination
Peptic ulcer	Burning or gnawing pain	May have epigastric tenderness on palpation
Gastritis	Constant burning pain in epigastrium	May be accompanied by nausea, vomiting, diarrhea or fever. Physical examination negative

Differential Diagnosis of Urinary Incontinence

Condition	History	Physical Findings
Stress incontinence	Small-volume incontinence with coughing, sneezing, laughing, running; history of prior pelvic surgery	Pelvic floor relaxation; cystocele, rectocele; lax urethral sphincter; loss of urine with provocative testing; atrophic vaginitis; postvoid residual <100 mL
Urge incontinence	Uncontrolled urge to void; large-volume incontinence; history of central nervous system (CNS) disorders such as stroke, multiple sclerosis, parkinsonism	Unexpected findings only as related to CNS disorder; postvoid residual <100 mL
Overflow incontinence	Small-volume incontinence, dribbling, hesitancy; in men symptoms of enlarged prostate—nocturia, dribbling, hesitancy decreased force and caliber of stream	Distended bladder; prostate hypertrophy; stool in rectum, fecal impaction; postvoid residual >100 mL
Functional incontinence	In neurogenic bladder—history of bowel problems, spinal cord injury, or multiple sclerosis Change in mental status, impaired mobility, new environment Medications—hypnotics, diuretics, anticholinergic agents, α-adrenergic agents, calcium channel blockers	Evidence of spinal cord disease or diabetic neuropathy; lax sphincter; gait disturbance Impaired mental status; impaired mobility Impaired mental status or unexpected findings only as related to other physical conditions

PEDIATRIC VARIATIONS

EXAMINATION

TECHNIQUE	FINDINGS

Inspect abdomen in all four quadrants

Infant's abdomen should be examined, if possible, during a time of relaxation and quiet. Sucking on a bottle or pacifier may help to relax infant.

■ *Contour/symmetry* **EXPECTED:** Until the age of 3 years, children's abdomens will protrude when standing.

■ *Surface motion* **EXPECTED:** Pulsation in epigastric area in infants.
UNEXPECTED: Peristaltic waves associated with pyloric stenosis.

Percuss abdomen

■ *Tone* **EXPECTED:** More tympany is present in children than adults.

Deeply palpate abdomen

■ *Umbilical ring* **EXPECTED:** Children up to 4 years old may have an umbilical hernia.

■ *Liver* **EXPECTED:** Liver may be palpable in young children 2 to 3 cm below costal margin.

Age	Liver Span (cm)
6 months	2.4-2.8
12 months	2.8-3.1
24 months	3.5-3.6
3 years	4.0
4 years	4.3-4.4
5 years	4.5-5.1
6 years	4.8-5.1
8 years	5.1-5.6
10 years	5.5-6.1

SAMPLE DOCUMENTATION

Subjective. A 44-year-old female complains of burning sensation in epigastric area and chest. Occurs after eating, especially with spicy foods. Lasts 1 to 2 hours and is worse when lying down. Sometimes causes bitter taste in mouth. Also feels bloated. Antacids do not relieve symptoms. Denies nausea/vomiting/diarrhea. No cough or shortness of breath.

Objective. Abdomen rounded and symmetric, with white striae adjacent to umbilicus in all quadrants. A well-healed 5-cm white surgical scar evident in right lower quadrant. No areas of visible pulsations or peristalsis. Active bowel sounds audible. Percussion tones tympanic over epigastrium and resonant over remainder of abdomen. Liver span 8 cm at right midclavicular line. On inspiration, liver edge firm, smooth, nontender. No splenomegaly. Musculature soft and relaxed to light palpation. No masses or areas of tenderness to deep palpation. Superficial reflexes intact. No costovertebral angle tenderness.

FEMALE GENITALIA

EQUIPMENT

- Drapes
- Speculum
- Gloves
- Water-soluble lubricant
- Lamp or light source
- Specimen collection equipment such as:
  - Sterile cotton swabs
  - Glass slides
  - Wooden or plastic spatula
  - Cervical brush devices
  - Cytologic fixative
  - Culture plates or media, if needed
  - DNA probe kits for chlamydia and gonorrhea, if needed

EXAMINATION

Have patient in lithotomy position, draped for minimal exposure.

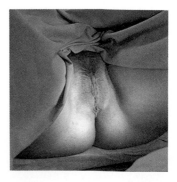

TECHNIQUE	FINDINGS

EXTERNAL GENITALIA

Wear gloves on both hands

Ask patient to separate or drop open her knees. Tell patient you are beginning the examination, then touch either lower thigh and—without breaking contact—move hand along thigh to external genitalia.

Inspect and palpate mons pubis

■ *Characteristics*

■ *Pubic hair*

EXPECTED: Skin smooth and clean.
UNEXPECTED: Improper hygiene.
EXPECTED: Regularly distributed female pubic hair.
UNEXPECTED: Nits or lice.

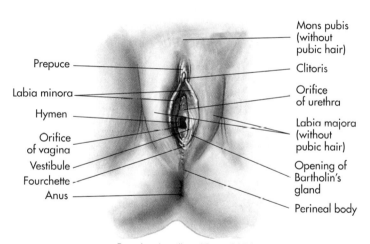

Mons pubis (without pubic hair)
Prepuce
Clitoris
Labia minora
Orifice of urethra
Hymen
Labia majora (without pubic hair)
Orifice of vagina
Vestibule
Fourchette
Opening of Bartholin's gland
Anus
Perineal body

From Lowdermilk and Perry, 2004.

Inspect and palpate labia

■ *Labia majora*

EXPECTED: Gaping or closed, dry or moist, shriveled or full, tissue soft and homogeneous, usually symmetric.
UNEXPECTED: Swelling, redness, tenderness, discoloration, varicosities,

TECHNIQUE	**FINDINGS**
	obvious stretching, or signs of trauma or scarring. If excoriation, rashes, or lesions are present, ask patient whether she has been scratching.
▪ *Labia minora* Separate labia majora with fingers of one hand. With other hand, palpate labia minora between thumb and second finger.	**EXPECTED:** Moist, dark pink inner surface. Tissue soft and homogeneous. **UNEXPECTED:** Tenderness, inflammation, irritation, excoriation, caking of discharge in tissue folds, discoloration, ulcers, vesicles, irregularities, or nodules. Hyperemia of fourchette not related to recent sexual activity.

Inspect clitoris

▪ *Size and length*	**EXPECTED:** Length 2 cm or less; diameter 0.5 cm. **UNEXPECTED:** Enlargement, atrophy, inflammation, or adhesions.

Inspect urethral meatus and vaginal opening

▪ *Urethral orifice*	**EXPECTED:** Slit or irregular opening, close to or in vaginal introitus, usually midline. **UNEXPECTED:** Discharge, polyps, caruncles, fistulas, lesions, irritation, inflammation, or dilation.
▪ *Vaginal introitus*	**EXPECTED:** Thin vertical slit or large orifice with irregular edges. Tissue moist. **UNEXPECTED:** Swelling, discoloration, discharge, lesions, fistulas, or fissures.

Milk Skene glands

Tell patient you will be inserting one finger into her vagina and pressing forward with it. With	**UNEXPECTED:** Discharge or tenderness. Note color, consistency, odor of any

TECHNIQUE	FINDINGS

palm up, insert index finger to second joint, press upward, and milk Skene glands by moving finger outward. Perform on both sides of urethra and directly on urethra.

discharge; obtain culture.

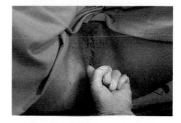

Palpate Bartholin glands

Tell patient she will feel you pressing around the entrance to her vagina. Palpate lateral tissue between index finger and thumb, then palpate entire area bilaterally, particularly posterolateral portion of labia majora.

EXPECTED: No swelling.
UNEXPECTED: Swelling, tenderness, masses, heat, fluctuation, or discharge. Note color, consistency, odor of any discharge; obtain culture.

Test vaginal muscle tone if indicated

Ask patient to squeeze vaginal opening around your finger.

EXPECTED: Fairly tight squeezing by some nulliparous women, less so by some multiparous women.
UNEXPECTED: Protrusion of cervix or uterus.

Locate the cervix

With your finger still in place you can reach in further to locate the cervix and note the direction in which it points. This may help you locate the cervix when you insert the speculum.

EXPECTED: Midline, may point horizontally, anteriorly or posteriorly.
UNEXPECTED: Deviates to right or left.

Inspect for bulging and urinary incontinence if indicated

Ask patient to bear down.

EXPECTED: No bulging.
UNEXPECTED: Bulging of anterior or posterior wall, or urinary incontinence.

TECHNIQUE	FINDINGS

Inspect and palpate perineum

Compress perineal tissue between finger and thumb.

EXPECTED: Perineum surface smooth—generally thick and smooth in a nulliparous woman, thinner and rigid in a multiparous woman. Possible episiotomy scarring in women who have borne children.
UNEXPECTED: Tenderness, inflammation, fistulas, lesions, or growths.

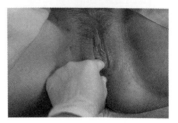

Inspect anus

■ *Skin characteristics*

EXPECTED: Skin darkly pigmented and possibly coarse.
UNEXPECTED: Scarring, lesions, inflammation, fissures, lumps, skin tags, or excoriation.

INTERNAL GENITALIA—SPECULUM EXAMINATION

If you touched the perineum or anal skin while examining the external genitalia, change gloves before beginning internal examination.

Lubricate speculum and gloved fingers with water or water-soluble gel lubricant. Water is preferred if obtaining a Pap smear.

Insert speculum

Tell patient she will feel you touching her again, then insert two fingers of hand not holding the speculum just inside vaginal introitus and gently press downward. Ask patient to breathe slowly and try to consciously relax her muscles.

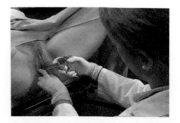

TECHNIQUE	FINDINGS

Use fingers of that hand to separate labia minora widely so that the vaginal opening becomes clearly visible. Then slowly insert speculum along path of least resistance, often slightly downward, avoiding trauma to urethra and vaginal walls. Some clinicians insert speculum blades at an oblique angle; others prefer to keep blades horizontal. In either case avoid touching clitoris, catching pubic hair, or pinching labial skin. Insert speculum the length of the vaginal canal. Maintaining downward pressure, open speculum by pressing on thumb piece. Sweep speculum slowly upward until cervix comes into view. Adjust light, then manipulate speculum farther into vagina so that cervix is well exposed between anterior and posterior blades. Stabilize distal spread of blades, and adjust proximal spread as needed.

Inspect cervix

■ *Color*

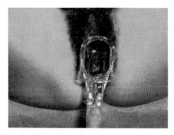

From Edge and Miller, 1994.

EXPECTED: Evenly distributed pink. Symmetric, circumscribed erythema around os can be expected.
UNEXPECTED: Bluish, pale, or reddened cervix (especially if

TECHNIQUE	**FINDINGS**
	patchy or with irregular borders).
▨ *Position*	**EXPECTED:** In midline, horizontal or pointing anteriorly or posteriorly. Protruding into vagina 1 to 3 cm. **UNEXPECTED:** Deviation to right or left. Protrusion into vagina greater than 1 to 3 cm.
▨ *Size*	**EXPECTED:** 3 cm in diameter. **UNEXPECTED:** Larger than 3 cm.
▨ *Shape*	**EXPECTED:** Uniform. **UNEXPECTED:** Distorted.
▨ *Surface characteristics*	**EXPECTED:** Surface smooth. Possible symmetric, reddened circle around os (squamocolumnar epithelium). Possible small, white, or yellow, raised round areas on cervix (nabothian cysts). **UNEXPECTED** Friable tissue, red patchy areas, granular areas, or white patches.
▨ *Discharge* Note any discharge. Determine origin—cervix or vagina.	**EXPECTED:** Odorless, creamy or clear, thick, thin, or stringy (often heavier at midcycle or immediately before menstruation). **UNEXPECTED:** Odorous and white to yellow, green, or gray.
▨ *Size and shape of os* Follow standard precautions for safe collection of human secretions.	**EXPECTED:** *Nulliparous woman:* Small, round, oval. *Multiparous woman:* Usually a horizontal slit or irregular and stellate. **UNEXPECTED:** Slit resulting from trauma from induced abortion, difficult removal of intrauterine device (IUD), or sexual abuse.

TECHNIQUE	FINDINGS

Withdraw speculum, and inspect vaginal walls

Unlock speculum, and remove it slowly, rotating it so vaginal walls can be inspected. Maintain downward pressure, and hook index finger over anterior blade as it is removed. Note odor of any discharge pooled in posterior blade, and obtain specimen if not already obtained.

EXPECTED: Vaginal wall color same pink as cervix or lighter; moist, smooth or rugated; and homogeneous. Thin, clear or cloudy, odorless secretions.

UNEXPECTED: Reddened patches, lesions, pallor, cracks, bleeding, nodules, swelling. Secretions that are profuse; thick, curdy, or frothy; gray, green, or yellow; or malodorous.

INTERNAL GENITALIA—BIMANUAL EXAMINATION

Change gloves, and then lubricate index and middle fingers of examining hand.

Tell patient you are going to examine her internally with your fingers. Prevent thumb from touching clitoris during examination.

Obtaining Vaginal Smears and Cultures

Vaginal specimens are obtained while the speculum is in place in the vagina but after the cervix and its surrounding tissue have been inspected. Collect specimens as indicated for a Papanicolaou (Pap) smear, sexually transmitted disease screening, and wet mount. Label the specimen with the patient's name and a description of the specimen (e.g., cervical smear, vaginal smear, and culture). Be sure to follow standard precautions for the safe collection of human secretions.

Pap Smear

Brushes and brooms are now being used in conjunction with, or instead of, the conventional spatula to improve the quality of cells obtained. The cylindric-type brush (e.g., a Cytobrush) collects endocervical cells only. First, collect a sample from the ectocervix with a spatula. Insert the longer projection of the spatula into the cervical os. Rotate it 360 degrees, keeping it flush against the cervical tissue. Withdraw the spatula, and spread the specimen on a glass

Continued

Obtaining Vaginal Smears and Cultures—cont'd

slide. A single light stroke with each side of the spatula is sufficient to thin out the specimen over the slide. Fix the specimen and label as ectocervical. Then introduce the brush device into the vagina, and insert it into the cervical os until only the bristles closest to the handle are exposed. Slowly rotate one half to one full turn. Remove and prepare the endocervical smear by rolling the brush with moderate pressure across a glass slide. Fix the specimen and label as endocervical. Alternatively, both specimens can be placed on a single slide.

The broom-type brush is used for collecting both ectocervical and endocervical cells at the same time. The broom has flexible plastic bristles, which are reported to cause less blood spotting after the examination. Introduce the brush into the vagina, and insert the central long bristles into the cervical os until the lateral bristles bend fully against the ectocervix. Maintain gentle pressure, and rotate the brush by rolling the handle between the thumb and forefinger three to five times to the left and right. Withdraw the brush, and transfer the sample to a glass slide with two single "paint" strokes. Apply first one side of the bristle, then turn the brush over, and paint the slide again in exactly the same area. Apply fixative and label as the

ectocervical and endocervical specimen.

For the liquid preparation technology, using the broom-type device, insert the central bristles of the broom into the endocervical canal deep enough to allow the shorter bristles to fully contact the ectocervix. Push gently, and rotate the broom clockwise **five** times. Rinse the broom into the solution vial by pushing the broom into the bottom of the vial 10 times, forcing the bristles apart. As a final step, swirl the broom vigorously to further release material. Discard the collection device. Alternatively, deposit the broom end of the device directly into the collection vial. With any collection device, be sure to follow the manufacturer's and laboratory instructions to collect and preserve the specimen appropriately. Close the vial tightly to prevent leakage and loss of the sample during transport.

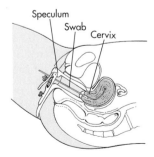

Speculum

Swab

Cervix

Gonococcal Culture Specimen

Immediately after the Pap smear is obtained, introduce a sterile cotton swab into the vagina, and insert it into the cervical os. Hold it in place for 10 to 30 seconds. Withdraw the swab, and spread the specimen in a large Z pattern over the culture medium, rotating the swab at the same time. Label the tube or plate, and follow agency routine for transporting and warming the specimen. If indicated, an anal culture can be obtained after the vaginal speculum has been removed. Insert a fresh, sterile cotton swab about 2.5 cm into the rectum, and rotate it in a full circle. Hold it in place for 10 to 30 seconds. Withdraw the swab, and prepare the specimen as described for the vaginal culture. Gonococcal cultures are now used less frequently than the combined DNA probe for chlamydia and gonorrhea.

DNA Probe for Chlamydia and Gonorrhea

This test involves the construction of a nucleic acid sequence (called a probe) that will match a sequence in the DNA or RNA of the target tissue. Results are rapid and sensitive. Use a Dacron swab (with a plastic or wire shaft) when collecting the specimen; wooden, cotton-tipped applicators may interfere with test results. Also be sure to check the expiration date so as not to use out-of-date materials. Insert the swab into the cervical os, and rotate the swab in the endocervical canal for 30 seconds to ensure adequate sampling and absorption by the swab. Avoid contact with the vaginal mucous membranes, which would contaminate the specimen. Remove the swab, and place it in the tube containing the specimen reagent.

Wet Mount and Potassium Hydroxide (KOH) Procedures

In a woman with vaginal discharge, these microscope examinations can demonstrate the presence of *Trichomonas vaginalis,* bacterial vaginosis, or candidiasis. For the wet mount, obtain a specimen of vaginal discharge using a swab. Smear the sample on a glass slide, and add a drop of normal saline solution. Place a coverslip on the slide, and view under the microscope. The presence of trichomonads indicates *T. vaginalis.* The presence of bacteria-filled epithelial cells (clue cells) indicates bacterial vaginosis. On a separate glass slide, place a specimen of vaginal discharge, apply a drop of aqueous 10% KOH, and put a coverslip in place. The presence of a fishy odor (the "whiff test") suggests bacterial vaginosis. The KOH dissolves epithelial cells and debris and facilitates visualization of the mycelia of a fungus. View under the microscope for the presence of mycelial fragments, hypha, and budding yeast cells, which indicate candidiasis.

TECHNIQUE	FINDINGS

Palpate vaginal wall while inserting fingers into vagina

Insert tips of index and middle fingers into vaginal opening and press downward, waiting for muscles to relax. Gradually insert fingers full length while palpating vaginal wall.

EXPECTED: Smooth and homogeneous.
UNEXPECTED: Tenderness, lesions, cysts, nodules, masses, or growths.

Palpate cervix

Locate cervix with palmar surface of fingers, feel end, and run fingers around circumference to feel fornices.

■ *Size, shape, length*

EXPECTED: Consistent with speculum examination.

■ *Consistency*

EXPECTED: Firm in nonpregnant woman; softer in pregnant woman.
UNEXPECTED: Nodules, hardness, or roughness.

■ *Position*

EXPECTED: In midline horizontal or pointing anteriorly or posteriorly. Protruding into vagina 1 to 3 cm.
UNEXPECTED: Deviation to right or left. Protrusion into vagina greater than 1 to 3 cm.

■ *Mobility*
Grasp cervix gently between fingers and move from side to side. Observe patient's facial expression.

EXPECTED: 1 to 2 cm movement in each direction. Minimal discomfort.
UNEXPECTED: Pain on movement ("cervical motion tenderness").

Palpate uterus

■ *Location and position*
Place palmar surface of outside hand on abdominal midline, halfway between umbilicus and symphysis pubis, and place intravaginal fingers in anterior fornix.

EXPECTED: In midline, horizontal, or pointing anteriorly or posteriorly. Protruding into vagina 1 to 3 cm.
UNEXPECTED: Deviation to right or left. Protrusion into vagina greater than 1 to 3 cm.

TECHNIQUE

FINDINGS

As shown in figure at right, slowly slide outside hand toward pubis while pressing down and forward with flat surface of fingers; at the same time, push inward and up with fingertips of intravaginal hand while pushing down on cervix with backs of fingers. If uterus is anteverted or anteflexed, you should feel fundus between fingers of two hands at level of pubis.

If uterus cannot be felt with this maneuver, place intravaginal fingers together in posterior fornix and outside hand immediately above symphysis pubis. Press firmly down with outside hand while pressing inward against cervix with intravaginal hand. If uterus is retroverted or retroflexed, you should feel fundus. If uterus cannot be felt with either of these maneuvers, move intravaginal fingers to each side of cervix, and while keeping contact with cervix, press inward and feel as far as possible. Slide fingers so they are on top and bottom of cervix and continue pressing in while moving fingers to feel as much of uterus as possible (when uterus is in midposition, you will not be able to feel it with outside hand).

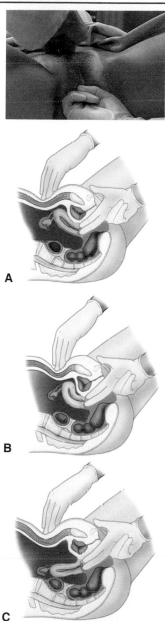

A

B

C

A, Anteverted. **B,** Anteflexed.
C, Retroverted.

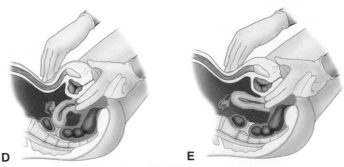

D, Retroflexed. **E,** Midposition of uterus.

■ *Size, shape, contour*

EXPECTED: Pear-shaped and 5.5 to 8.0 cm long (larger in all dimensions in multiparous women). Contour rounded and, in nonpregnant women, walls firm and smooth.
UNEXPECTED: Larger than expected or interrupted contour or smoothness.

■ *Mobility*
Gently move uterus between intravaginal fingers and outside hand.

EXPECTED: Mobile in anteroposterior plane.
UNEXPECTED: Fixed uterus or tenderness on movement.

Palpate ovaries

Place fingers of outside hand on lower right quadrant. With intravaginal hand facing up, place both fingers in right lateral fornix. Press intravaginal fingers deeply in and up toward abdominal hand, while sweeping flat surface of fingers of outside hand deeply in and obliquely down toward symphysis pubis. Palpate entire area by firmly pressing outside hand and intravaginal fingers together. Repeat on left side.

TECHNIQUE	FINDINGS
■ *Consistency*	**EXPECTED:** If palpable, ovaries should feel firm, smooth, slightly to moderately tender. **UNEXPECTED:** Marked tenderness or nodularity. Palpable fallopian tubes.
■ *Size*	**EXPECTED:** About $3 \times 2 \times 1$ cm. **UNEXPECTED:** Enlargement.
■ *Shape*	**EXPECTED:** Ovoid.

Palpate adnexal areas

Use hand positions for palpating ovaries.	**EXPECTED:** Adnexa difficult to palpate. **UNEXPECTED:** Masses and tenderness. If adnexal masses are found, characterize by size, shape, location, consistency, tenderness.

INTERNAL GENITALIA—RECTOVAGINAL EXAMINATION

Change gloves. This examination may be uncomfortable for the patient. Assure her that although she may feel the urgency of a bowel movement, she will not have one. Ask her to breathe slowly and try to relax her sphincter, rectum, buttocks.

Insert index finger into vagina and middle finger into anus

To insert middle finger into anus, press against anus and ask patient to bear down. As she does, slip tip of finger into rectum just past sphincter.

Assess sphincter tone

Palpate area of anorectal junction and just above it. Ask patient to tighten and relax anal sphincter.	**EXPECTED:** Even sphincter tightening. **UNEXPECTED:** Extremely tight, lax, or absent sphincter.

Palpate anterior rectal wall and rectovaginal septum

Slide both fingers in as far as possible, then ask patient to	**EXPECTED:** Smooth and uninterrupted. Uterine body and

TECHNIQUE	FINDINGS
bear down. Rotate rectal finger to explore anterior rectal wall and palpate rectovaginal septum.	uterine fundus sometimes felt with retroflexed uterus. **UNEXPECTED:** Masses, polyps, nodules, strictures, irregularities, tenderness.

Palpate posterior aspect of uterus

Place outside hand just above symphysis pubis and press firmly and deeply down, while positioning intravaginal finger in posterior vaginal fornix and pressing strongly upward against posterior side of cervix, as shown in figure below. Palpate as much of posterior side of uterus as possible.	**EXPECTED:** Consistent with bimanual examination regarding location, position, size, shape, contour. **UNEXPECTED:** Tenderness.

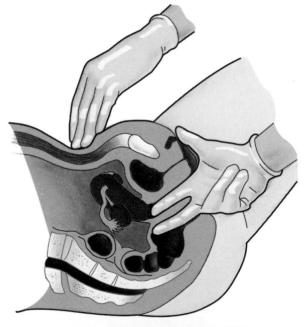

From Lowdermilk and Perry, 2004.

TECHNIQUE	FINDINGS

Palpate posterior rectal wall

As you withdraw fingers, rotate intrarectal finger to evaluate posterior rectal wall.

EXPECTED: Smooth and uninterrupted.

UNEXPECTED: Masses, polyps, nodules, strictures, irregularities, tenderness.

Note characteristics of feces when gloved finger removed

EXPECTED: Light to dark brown.

UNEXPECTED: Blood. Note color and prepare specimen for fecal occult blood testing (FOBT) if indicated

Wipe patient's perineum, using front-to-back stroke and clean tissue for each stroke

AIDS TO DIFFERENTIAL DIAGNOSIS

ABNORMALITY	DESCRIPTION
Premenstrual syndrome (PMS)	Edema, headache, weight gain, behavior disturbances such as irritability, nervousness, dysphoria, lack of coordination. Symptoms occur 5 to 7 days before menses, then subside.
Endometriosis	Pelvic pain, dysmenorrhea, heavy or prolonged menstrual flow.
Condyloma acuminatum (genital warts)	Warty lesions on labia, within vestibule, or in perianal region. Growths (generally whitish-pink to reddish-brown, discrete, soft) may occur singly or in clusters and may enlarge to cauliflower masses.
Herpes lesions	Small, red vesicles that may itch and usually are painful. Initial infection often extensive; recurrent infection normally a localized patch on vulva, perineum, vagina, or cervix.

ABNORMALITY	DESCRIPTION
Vaginal infections	Often vaginal discharge, possibly accompanied by urinary symptoms. Sometimes asymptomatic (see table on pp. 181–182).
Cervical carcinoma	Hard granular surface at or near cervical os. Lesion can evolve to form extensive, irregular, easily bleeding cauliflower growth. Precancerous and early cancer changes are detected by Pap smear, not by physical examination.
Uterine bleeding	See table on p. 183.
Pelvic inflammatory disease (PID)	*Acute PID:* Very tender bilateral adnexal areas. *Chronic PID:* Bilateral tender, irregular, fairly fixed adnexal areas.

Differential Diagnosis of Vaginal Discharges and Infections

Condition	History	Physical Findings	Diagnostic Tests
Physiologic vaginitis	Increase in discharge; no foul odor, itching, or edema	Clear or mucoid discharge; pH < 4.5	Wet mount: up to 3-5 white blood cells (WBCs); epithelial cells
Bacterial vaginosis (Gardnerella vaginalis)	Foul-smelling discharge; complains of "fishy odor"	Homogeneous, thin, white or gray discharge; pH > 4.5	+ KOH "whiff" test; wet mount: + clue cells
Candida vulvovaginitis (Candida albicans)	Pruritic discharge, itching of labia; itching may extend to thighs	White, curdy discharge; pH 4.0-5.0; cervix may be red; may have erythema of perineum and thighs	KOH prep: mycelia, budding, branching yeast, pseudohyphae
Trichomoniasis (Trichomonas vaginalis)	Watery discharge; foul odor; dysuria and dyspareunia with severe infection	Profuse, frothy, greenish discharge; pH 5.0-6.6; red, friable cervix with petechiae ("strawberry" cervix)	Wet mount: round or pear-shaped protozoa, motile "gyrating" flagella
Gonorrhea (Neisseria gonorrhoeae)	Partner with sexually transmitted disease; often asymptomatic or may have symptoms of pelvic inflammatory disease	Purulent discharge from cervix; Skene/Bartholin gland inflammation; cervix and vulva may be inflamed	Gram stain, culture, DNA probe
Chlamydia (Chlamydia trachomatis)	Partner with nongonococcal urethritis; often asymptomatic; may complain of spotting after intercourse or urethritis	+/- purulent discharge; cervix may or may not be red or friable	DNA probe

Continued

Differential Diagnosis of Vaginal Discharges and Infections—cont'd

Condition	History	Physical Findings	Diagnostic Tests
Atrophic vaginitis	Dyspareunia; vaginal dryness; perimenopausal or postmenopausal	Pale, thin vaginal mucosa; pH > 4.5	Wet mount: folded, clumped epithelial cells
Allergic vaginitis	New bubble bath, soap, douche, or other hygiene products	Foul smell, erythema; pH < 4.5	Wet mount: WBCs
Foreign body	Red and swollen vulva; vaginal discharge; history of tampon, condom, or diaphragm use	Bloody or foul-smelling discharge	Wet mount: WBCs

Bacterial vaginosis

Candida vulvovaginitis

Trichomoniasis

Types of Uterine Bleeding and Associated Causes

Type	Common Causes
Midcycle spotting	Midcycle estradiol fluctuation associated with ovulation
Delayed menstruation	Anovulation or threatened abortion with excessive bleeding
Frequent bleeding	Chronic pelvic inflammatory disease, endometriosis, dysfunctional uterine bleeding (DUB), anovulation
Profuse menstrual bleeding	Endometrial polyps, DUB, adenomyosis, submucous leiomyomas, intrauterine device
Intermenstrual or irregular bleeding	Endometrial polyps, DUB, uterine or cervical cancer, oral contraceptives
Postmenopausal bleeding	Endometrial hyperplasia, estrogen therapy, endometrial cancer

Modified from Thompson et al, 1997.

PEDIATRIC VARIATIONS

EXAMINATION

TECHNIQUE	**FINDINGS**
Inspect external genitalia	
Examine infant using the frog-leg position.	**EXPECTED:** Genitalia of newborn reflects influence of maternal hormones. Labia majora and minora may be swollen, with labia minora often more prominent.
Inspect clitoris	
■ *Size and length*	**EXPECTED:** The clitoris of a term infant is usually covered by labia minora and may appear relatively large.
Inspect urethral meatus and vaginal opening	
■ *Inspect for discharge in infants and children*	**EXPECTED:** Mucoid whitish vaginal discharge is frequently seen during newborn period and sometimes as late as 4 weeks after birth. Discharge may be mixed with blood.

TECHNIQUE	FINDINGS
	UNEXPECTED: Mucoid discharge from irritation by diapers or powder; any discharge in children.

Assess pubertal development

Assess Tanner stages of female pubic hair development.

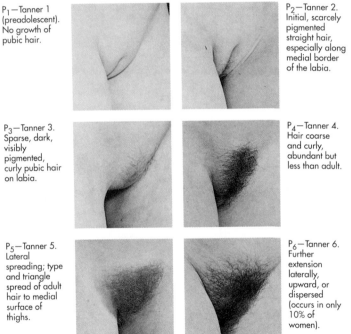

P₁—Tanner 1 (preadolescent). No growth of pubic hair.

P₂—Tanner 2. Initial, scarcely pigmented straight hair, especially along medial border of the labia.

P₃—Tanner 3. Sparse, dark, visibly pigmented, curly pubic hair on labia.

P₄—Tanner 4. Hair coarse and curly, abundant but less than adult.

P₅—Tanner 5. Lateral spreading; type and triangle spread of adult hair to medial surface of thighs.

P₆—Tanner 6. Further extension laterally, upward, or dispersed (occurs in only 10% of women).

Six stages of pubic hair development in females. *From Van Wieringen et al, 1971. Reprinted by permission of Kluwer Academic Publishers.*

"Red Flags" for Sexual Abuse

The following signs and symptoms in children or adolescents should raise your suspicion for sexual abuse. Remember, however, that any sign or symptom by itself is of limited significance; it may be related to sexual abuse, or it may be from another cause altogether. This is an area in which good clinical judgment is imperative. Each sign or symptom must be considered in context with the particular child's health status, stage of growth and development, and entire history.

Medical complaints and findings
- Evidence of general physical abuse or neglect
- Evidence of trauma and/or scarring in genital, anal, and perianal areas
- Unusual changes in skin color or pigmentation in genital or anal area
- Presence of sexually transmitted disease (oral, anal, genital)
- Anorectal problems such as itching, bleeding, pain, fecal incontinence, poor anal sphincter tone, bowel habit dysfunction
- Genitourinary problems such as rash or sores in genital area, vaginal odor, pain (including abdominal pain), itching, bleeding, discharge, dysuria, hematuria, urinary tract infections, enuresis

Examples of nonspecific behavioral manifestations
- Problems with school
- Dramatic weight changes or eating disturbances
- Depression
- Sleep problems or nightmares
- Sudden change in personality or behavior
- Aggression or destructiveness
- Sudden avoidance of certain people or places

Examples of sexual behaviors that are concerning
- Use of sexually provocative mannerisms
- Excessive masturbation or sexual behavior that cannot be redirected
- Age-inappropriate sexual knowledge or experience
- Repeated object insertion into vagina and/or anus
- Child asking to be touched/kissed in genital area
- Sex play between children with 4 years or more age difference
- Sex play that involves the use of force, threats, or bribes

Modified from Koop, 1988; McClain et al, 2000; Hornor, 2004.

Early Signs of Pregnancy

Sign	Finding	Approximate Weeks of Gestation

Following are physical signs that occur early in pregnancy. These signs, along with internal ballottement, palpation of fetal parts, and positive test results for urine or serum human chorionic gonadotropin, are probable indicators of pregnancy. They are considered "probable" because clinical conditions other than pregnancy may cause any one of them. Their occurrence together, however, creates a strong case for the presence of a pregnancy.

Sign	Finding	Approximate Weeks of Gestation
Goodell	Softening of cervix	4-6
Hegar	Softening of uterine isthmus	6-8
McDonald	Easy flexing of fundus on cervix	7-8
Braun von Fernwald	Fullness and softening of fundus near site of implantation	7-8
Piskacek	Palpable lateral bulge or soft prominence of one uterine cornu	7-8
Chadwick	Bluish color of cervix, vagina, vulva	8-12

SAMPLE DOCUMENTATION

Subjective. A 45-year-old female with vaginal discharge and itching for past week. Has had yeast infections before. Completed course of antibiotics for sinusitis 2 days ago. Last menstrual period 2 weeks ago. Sexually active, one partner, mutually monogamous. No unusual vaginal bleeding. Does not douche.

Objective. *External:* Female hair distribution; no masses, lesions, or swelling. Urethral meatus intact without erythema or discharge. Perineum intact with healed episiotomy scar present. No lesions.

Internal: Vaginal mucosa pink and moist with rugae present. No unusual odors. Profuse thick, white, curdy discharge. Cervix pink with horizontal slit midline; no lesions or discharge.

Bimanual: Cervix smooth, firm, mobile. No cervical motion tenderness. Uterus midline, anteverted, firm, smooth, nontender; not enlarged. Ovaries not palpable. No adnexal tenderness.

Rectovaginal: Septum intact. Sphincter tone intact; anal ring smooth and intact. No masses or tenderness.

chapter 15

MALE GENITALIA

EQUIPMENT

- Gloves
- Penlight

EXAMINATION

Have patient lying or standing to start examination.

TECHNIQUE	FINDINGS
Wear gloves on both hands	
Inspect pubic hair	
■ *Characteristics*	**EXPECTED:** Coarser than scalp hair.
■ *Distribution*	**EXPECTED:** Male hair distribution. Abundant in pubic region, continuing around scrotum to anal orifice, possibly continuing in narrowing midline to umbilicus. Penis without hair, scrotum with scant hair **UNEXPECTED:** Alopecia.
Inspect glans penis	
■ *Uncircumcised patient* Retract foreskin or ask patient to do so.	**EXPECTED:** Dorsal vein apparent. Foreskin easily retracted. White, cheesy smegma visible over glans. **UNEXPECTED:** Tight foreskin (phimosis). Lesions or discharge.

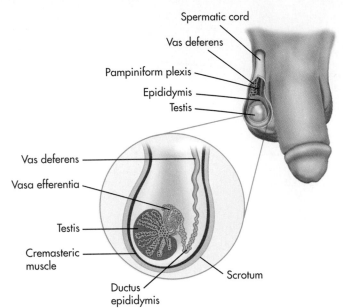

TECHNIQUE	FINDINGS
▪ *Circumcised patient*	**EXPECTED:** Dorsal vein apparent. Exposed glans erythematous and dry. **UNEXPECTED:** Lesions or discharge.

Examine external meatus of urethra (foreskin retracted in uncircumcised patient)

▪ *Shape*	**EXPECTED:** Slitlike opening. **UNEXPECTED:** Pinpoint or round opening.
▪ *Location*	**EXPECTED:** On ventral surface and only millimeters from tip of glans. **UNEXPECTED:** Any place other than tip of glans or along shaft of penis.
▪ *Urethral orifice* Press glans between thumb and forefinger.	**EXPECTED:** Opening glistening and pink. **UNEXPECTED:** Bright erythema or discharge.

TECHNIQUE	**FINDINGS**

Palpate penis

EXPECTED: Soft (flaccid penis).
UNEXPECTED: Tenderness, induration, or nodularity. Prolonged erection (priapism).

Strip urethra

Firmly compress base of penis with thumb and forefinger; move toward glans.

UNEXPECTED: Discharge.

Inspect scrotum and ventral surface of penis

▪ *Color*

EXPECTED: Darker than body skin and often reddened in red-haired patients.

▪ *Texture*

EXPECTED: Surface possibly coarse. Small lumps on scrotal skin (sebaceous or epidermoid cysts) that sometimes discharge oily material.

▪ *Shape*

EXPECTED: Asymmetry. Thickness varying with temperature, age, emotional state.
UNEXPECTED: Unusual thickening, often with pitting.

Palpate inguinal canal for direct or indirect hernia

With patient standing, ask him to bear down as if for bowel movement. While he strains, inspect area of inguinal canal and region of fossa ovalis.
Ask patient to relax, and insert examining finger into lower part of scrotum and carry upward along vas deferens into inguinal canal, as shown in figure on p. 190.
Ask patient to cough.
Repeat examination on opposite side.

EXPECTED: Presence of oval external ring.
UNEXPECTED: Feeling a viscus against examining finger with coughing. If hernia felt, note as indirect (felt within inguinal canal or even into scrotum) or direct (felt medial to external canal).

TECHNIQUE	FINDINGS

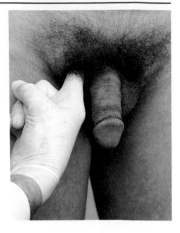

Palpate testes

Use thumb and first two fingers.

- *Consistency*

  EXPECTED: Smooth and rubbery. Sensitive to gentle compression.

  UNEXPECTED: Tenderness or nodules. Total insensitivity to painful stimuli.

- *Texture*

  UNEXPECTED: Irregular texture.

- *Size*

  UNEXPECTED: Irregular size; asymmetry in size, less than 1 cm or greater than 5 cm.

- *Descension*

  UNEXPECTED: Cryptorchidism.

Palpate epididymides

EXPECTED: Smooth and discrete, with larger part cephalad.

UNEXPECTED: Tenderness.

Palpate vas deferens

Palpate from testicle to inguinal ring. Repeat with other testicle.

EXPECTED: Smooth and discrete.

UNEXPECTED: Beaded or lumpy.

TECHNIQUE	FINDINGS

Palpate for inguinal lymph nodes

Ask patient to lie supine, with knee slightly flexed on side of palpation.

EXPECTED: Nodes unable to be palpated.
UNEXPECTED: Enlarged, tender, red or discolored, fixed, matted, inflamed, or warm nodes and increased vascularity.

Elicit cremasteric reflex bilaterally

Stroke inner thigh with blunt instrument. Repeat with other thigh.

AIDS TO DIFFERENTIAL DIAGNOSIS

ABNORMALITY	DESCRIPTION
Herpes	Superficial vesicles—located on glans, penile shaft, or base of penis—that are frequently quite painful. Often associated with inguinal lymphadenopathy and systemic symptoms (e.g., fever) in primary infection.
Hernia	See table on p. 192.
Hydrocele	Nontender, smooth, firm mass in scrotum. Transilluminates.
Varicocele	Abnormal tortuosity and dilated veins of pampiniform plexus within spermatic cord. Generally on left side and sometimes painful.
Epididymitis	Pain and possible erythema of overlying scrotum. Fever and white blood cells and bacteria in urine often accompany condition. In chronic form, epididymis feels firm and lumpy and may be slightly tender, and vasa deferentia may be beaded.
Priapism	Prolonged painful penile erection. May occur in patients with leukemia or sickle cell disease.

ABNORMALITY	DESCRIPTION
Hypospadias	Urethral meatus is located on ventral surface of glans, penile shaft, or perineal area.
Epispadias	Urethral meatus is located on dorsal surface of penile shaft.

Distinguishing Characteristics of Hernias

	Indirect Inguinal	Direct Inguinal	Femoral
Incidence	Most common type of hernia; both sexes are affected; often patients are children and young males	Less common than indirect inguinal; occurs more in males than females; more common in those older than 40 years	Least common type of hernia; occurs more often in females than males; rare in children
Occurrence	Through internal inguinal ring; can remain in canal, exit external ring, or pass into scrotum; may be bilateral	Through external inguinal ring; located in region of Hesselbach triangle; rarely enters scrotum	Through femoral ring, femoral canal, fossa ovalis
Presentation	Soft swelling in area of internal ring; pain on straining; hernia comes down canal and touches fingertip on examination	Bulge in area of Hesselbach triangle; usually painless; easily reduced; hernia bulges anteriorly, pushes against side of finger on examination	Right side presentation more common than left; pain may be severe; inguinal canal empty on examination

PEDIATRIC VARIATIONS

EXAMINATION

TECHNIQUE	FINDINGS

Inspect glans penis

- *Uncircumcised patient*
  Retract foreskin.

EXPECTED: In children, foreskin is fully retractable by age 3 to 4 years. Before that age, forced retraction of foreskin may result in injury.

Palpate scrotum

- *Descension*
  Palpate testes in children to determine whether testes have descended.
  If any mass other than testicles or spermatic cord is palpated in scrotum, determine whether it is filled with fluid, gas, or solid material.

EXPECTED: Bilaterally palpable; 1 cm. Considered descended if testis can be pushed into scrotum.

UNEXPECTED: If penlight transilluminates, most likely contains fluid (hydrocele). If no light transillumination, most likely a hernia.

Evaluate maturation in adolescence

Assess stage of pubertal development

In males, assess the stage of genital and pubic hair development.

EXPECTED: Tanner stages of male pubic hair and external genital development progress in the sequence shown on p. 194.

UNEXPECTED: Failure to mature and premature maturation.

G₁—Tanner 1. Testes, scrotum, and penis are the same size and shape as in the young child.

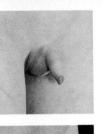

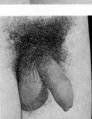

G₂—Tanner 2. Enlargement of scrotum and testes. The skin of the scrotum becomes redder, thinner, and wrinkled. Penis no larger or scarcely so.

G₃—Tanner 3. Enlargement of the penis, especially in length; further enlargement of testes; descent of scrotum.

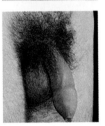

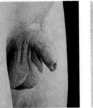

G₄—Tanner 4. Continued enlargement of the penis and sculpturing of the glans; increased pigmentation of scrotum. This stage is sometimes best

G₅—Tanner 5 (adult stage). Scrotum ample, penis reaching nearly to bottom of scrotum.

Five stages of penis and testes/scrotum development in males. *From Van Wieringen et al, 1971. Reprinted by permission of Kluwer Academic Publishers.*

SAMPLE DOCUMENTATION

Genitalia. Circumcised. Glans, penile shaft, contents of scrotal sac are intact without lesions or areas of induration. Urethral meatus patent on ventral surface at tip of glans. No discharge evident. Scrotal contents smooth without swelling, masses, or tenderness. Testes equal size. Inguinal areas are smooth; no masses or nodes palpable. Inguinal canals are free of masses, bulges. Cremasteric reflex elicited.

ANUS, RECTUM, AND PROSTATE

EQUIPMENT

- Gloves
- Water-soluble lubricant
- Light source
- Drapes
- Fecal occult blood testing materials if indicated

EXAMINATION

Have patient in knee-chest or left lateral position with hips and knees flexed, or standing with hips flexed and upper body supported by examining table. Drape patient appropriately.

TECHNIQUE	FINDINGS
Wear gloves on both hands	
Inspect and palpate sacrococcygeal and perianal area	
■ *Skin characteristics*	**EXPECTED:** Smooth and uninterrupted. **UNEXPECTED:** Lumps, rashes, tenderness, inflammation, excoriation, pilonidal dimpling, or tufts of hair.

Inspect anus

Spread patient's buttocks. Examine, using penlight or lamp if needed, with patient relaxed as well as with patient bearing down.

TECHNIQUE	FINDINGS
■ *Skin characteristics*	**EXPECTED:** Skin coarser and darker than on buttocks. **UNEXPECTED:** Skin lesions, skin tags or warts, external or internal hemorrhoids, fissures and fistulas, rectal prolapse, or polyps. Describe any irregularities and locate using clock referents (12 o'clock ventral midline/6 o'clock dorsal midline).

Inspect, palpate, assess sphincter tone

Put water-soluble lubricant on index or middle finger; press pad against anal opening, and ask patient to bear down to relax external sphincter. As relaxation occurs, slip tip of finger into anal canal, as shown in figure at right. (Assure patient that although he or she may feel the urgency of a bowel movement, it will not occur.) Ask patient to tighten external sphincter around finger.	**EXPECTED:** Even sphincter tightening. **UNEXPECTED:** Patient discomfort. Lax or extremely tight sphincter, tenderness.

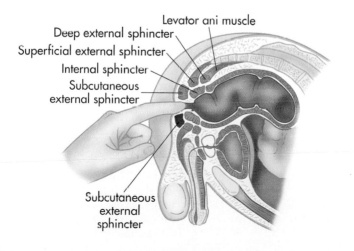

Levator ani muscle
Deep external sphincter
Superficial external sphincter
Internal sphincter
Subcutaneous external sphincter

Subcutaneous external sphincter

TECHNIQUE	FINDINGS

Palpate muscular anal ring

Rotate finger.

EXPECTED: Smooth, even with consistent pressure exerted.
UNEXPECTED: Nodules or other irregularities.

Palpate lateral and posterior rectal walls

Insert finger farther, and rotate to palpate lateral, then posterior, rectal walls. (If helpful, perform bidigital palpation with thumb and finger by lightly pressing thumb against perianal tissue and bringing finger toward thumb.)

EXPECTED: Smooth, even, uninterrupted.
UNEXPECTED: Nodules, masses, polyps, tenderness, or irregularities. (Internal hemorrhoids not ordinarily felt unless thrombosed.)

Males: Palpate posterior surface of prostate gland through anterior rectal wall

Rotate finger and palpate anterior rectal wall and posterior surface of prostate gland. (Alert patient that he may feel urge to urinate but will not.)

■ *Consistency and characteristics of anterior rectal wall*

EXPECTED: Smooth, even, uninterrupted.
UNEXPECTED: Nodules, masses, polyps, tenderness, or irregularities.

Consistency, contour, characteristics of prostate

EXPECTED: Surface firm and smooth, lateral lobes symmetric, median sulcus palpable, seminal vesicles not palpable.
UNEXPECTED: Rubberiness, bogginess, fluctuant softness, stony hard nodularity, tenderness, obliterated sulcus, or palpable seminal vesicles.

■ *Mobility of prostate gland*

EXPECTED: Slightly movable.

■ *Size of prostate gland*

EXPECTED: 4 cm diameter with less than 1 cm protruding into rectum.

TECHNIQUE	FINDINGS
	UNEXPECTED: Protrusion greater than 1 cm (note distance of protrusion). **UNEXPECTED:** Discharge that appears at urethral meatus (collect specimen for microscopic examination).

Females: Palpate uterus through anterior rectal wall

Attempt to palpate uterus and cervix through anterior rectal wall.

■ *Position*	**EXPECTED:** Midline, retroflexed or retroverted. **UNEXPECTED:** Deviation to right or left.
■ *Surface characteristics*	**EXPECTED:** Smooth. **UNEXPECTED:** Irregular.

Have patient bear down, and palpate deeper

Ask patient to bear down while you reach farther into rectum. *Females:* Explore in cul-de-sac. *Males:* Explore above prostate.

UNEXPECTED: Tenderness of peritoneal area or nodules.

Withdraw finger, and examine fecal material

■ *Color and consistency*	**EXPECTED:** Soft and brown. **UNEXPECTED:** Blood; pus; or light tan, gray, or tarry black stool. If indicated, fecal material can be tested for blood using a chemical guaiac procedure.

AIDS TO DIFFERENTIAL DIAGNOSIS

ABNORMALITY	DESCRIPTION
Anal warts (condyloma acuminata)	Pink to whitish growths on the anus and genitalia; caused by infection with the human papilloma virus (HPV). First appear as painless tiny blemishes that, left untreated, become larger and more numerous.

ABNORMALITY	DESCRIPTION
	Transmitted by direct sexual contact.
Perianal and perirectal abscesses	Pain and tenderness in anal area, usually accompanied by a fever.
Enterobius infestation in children	Intense perianal itching, especially at night.
Anorectal fissure and fistula	*Fissure:* Pain, itching, or bleeding, with spastic internal sphincter. *Fistula:* Elevated, red, granular tissue at external opening, possibly with serosanguineous or purulent drainage on compression of the area.
Hemorrhoids	*External:* Itching and bleeding with defecation. Thrombosed hemorrhoids appear as blue, shiny masses at anus. *Internal:* Bleeding with or without defecation. Do not cause discomfort unless thrombosed, prolapsed, or infected.
Rectal carcinoma	Generally asymptomatic.
Prostatic carcinoma	On rectal examination, a hard irregular nodule may be palpable. Prostate feels asymmetric and median sulcus is obliterated in advanced carcinoma.
Prostatitis	In acute prostatitis the prostate is enlarged, acutely tender, and often asymmetric. May have urethral discharge and fever. Chronic prostatitis usually asymptomatic; however, the prostate may feel boggy, enlarged, and tender or have palpable areas of fibrosis.
Benign prostatic hypertrophy	Hesitancy on urination, decreased force and caliber of stream, dribbling, incomplete emptying of bladder, nocturia, dysuria.

Prostate Enlargement

Prostate enlargement is classified by the amount of protrusion into the rectum:

Grade I:	1 to 2 cm
Grade II:	2 to 3 cm
Grade III:	3 to 4 cm
Grade IV:	More than 4 cm

PEDIATRIC VARIATIONS

EXAMINATION

TECHNIQUE	FINDINGS
Examine the patency of the anus and its position in all newborn infants. To determine patency, insert a lubricated catheter no more than 1 cm into the rectum.	**EXPECTED:** Catheter inserts; patency confirmed by passage of meconium **UNEXPECTED:** Not able to insert catheter; no evidence of stool
Inspect perianal area	**UNEXPECTED:** Parental complaints of infant's or child's irritability at night or evidence that child has itching in perianal area may indicate presence of parasites such as roundworms or pinworms. Specimen collection and microscopic examination are necessary to confirm findings.

TECHNIQUE	FINDINGS
	Shrunken buttocks suggest a chronic debilitating disease. Asymmetric creases occur with congenital dislocation of the hips. Perirectal redness and irritation are suggestive of pinworms, *Candida,* or other irritants of the diaper area. Rectal prolapse results from constipation, diarrhea, or sometimes severe coughing or straining. Hemorrhoids are rare in children, and their presence suggests a serious underlying problem such as portal hypertension. Small, flat flaps of skin around the rectum (condylomas) may be syphilitic in origin. Sinuses, tufts of hair, and dimpling in the pilonidal area may indicate lower spinal deformities.

SAMPLE DOCUMENTATION

Subjective. A 57-year-old male complains of nighttime urination for the past several months, at least twice per night. Restricts fluid intake after 8 PM. Notices difficulty in starting stream. No pain or bleeding on urination. No change in caliber of stream. Denies change in bowel habits or stool characteristics. No history of prostatitis or enlarged prostate.

Objective. Perianal area intact without lesions or visible hemorrhoids. An external skin tag is visible in the 6 o'clock position. No fissures or fistulas. Sphincter tightens evenly. Prostate is symmetric, smooth, boggy, with 1-cm protrusion into rectum. Medial sulcus present. Nontender, no nodules. Rectal walls free of masses. Moderate amount of soft stool present; occult blood test result negative.

MUSCULOSKELETAL SYSTEM

EQUIPMENT

- Goniometer
- Skin-marking pencil
- Reflex hammer
- Tape measure

EXAMINATION

Begin examination as patient enters rooms, observing gait and posture. During examination, note ease of movement when patient walks, sits, rises, takes off garments, responds to directions.

TECHNIQUE	FINDINGS

POSTURE AND GENERAL GUIDELINES

Inspect skeleton and extremities, comparing sides

Inspect anterior, posterior, lateral aspects of posture; ability to stand erect; body parts; extremities.

- *Size, alignment, contour, symmetry*
  Measure extremities when lack of symmetry is noted in length or circumference

EXPECTED: Bilateral symmetry of length, circumference, alignment, position and number of skin folds; symmetric body parts; and aligned extremities.
UNEXPECTED: Gross deformity, lordosis, kyphosis, scoliosis, bony enlargement.

TECHNIQUE   **FINDINGS**

Inspect skin and subcutaneous tissues over muscles, cartilage, bones, joints

UNEXPECTED: Discoloration, swelling, or masses.

Inspect muscles, and compare sides

■ *Size and symmetry*
EXPECTED: Approximately symmetric bilateral muscle size.
UNEXPECTED: Gross hypertrophy or atrophy, fasciculations, or spasms.

Palpate all bones, joints, surrounding muscles (palpate inflamed joints last)

■ *Muscle tone*
EXPECTED: Firm.
UNEXPECTED: Hard or doughy, spasticity.

■ *Characteristics*
UNEXPECTED: Heat, tenderness, swelling, fluctuation of a joint, synovial thickening, crepitus, resistance to pressure, or discomfort to pressure on bones and joints.

Test each major joint and related muscle groups for active and passive range of motion, and compare sides

Ask patient to move each joint through range of motion (see instructions for specific joints and muscles in individual sections that follow), then ask patient to relax as you passively move same joints until end of range is felt.

EXPECTED: Passive range of motion often exceeds active range of motion by 5 degrees. Range of motion with passive and active maneuvers should be equal between contralateral joints.
UNEXPECTED: Pain, limitation of motion, spastic movement, joint instability, deformity, contracture, discrepancies greater than 5 degrees between active and passive range of motion. When increase or limitation in range of motion is found, measure angles

TECHNIQUE	FINDINGS

of greatest flexion and extension with goniometer, as shown in figure below, and compare with values as described for specific joints in individual extremities.

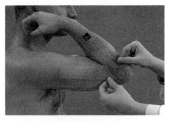

Goniometer

Test major muscle groups for strength, and compare contralateral sides

For each muscle group, ask patient to contract a muscle by flexing or extending a joint and to resist as you apply opposing force. Compare bilaterally.

EXPECTED: Bilaterally symmetric strength with full resistance to opposition.
UNEXPECTED: Inability to produce full resistance. Grade muscular strength according to table below.

TEMPOROMANDIBULAR JOINT

Palpate joint space for clicking, popping, pain

Locate temporomandibular joints with fingertips placed just anterior to tragus of each ear, as shown in

EXPECTED: Audible or palpable snapping or clicking may be noted.

Muscle Strength Assessment

Muscle Function Level	Grade
No evidence of contractility	0
Slight contractility, no movement	1
Full range of motion, gravity eliminated*	2
Full range of motion against gravity	3
Full range of motion against gravity, some resistance	4
Full range of motion against gravity, full resistance	5

From Jacobson, 1998.
*Passive movement.

TECHNIQUE	FINDINGS
figure at right. Ask patient to open mouth and allow fingertips to slip into joint space. Gently palpate.	**UNEXPECTED:** Pain, crepitus, locking, or popping.

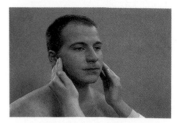

Palpating temporomandibular joint

Test range of motion

Ask patient to:

- *Open and close mouth* — **EXPECTED:** Opens 3 to 6 cm between upper and lower teeth.
- *Move jaw laterally to each side* — **EXPECTED:** Mandible moves 1 to 2 cm in each direction.
- *Protrude and retract jaw* — **EXPECTED:** Both protrusion and retraction possible.

Test strength of temporalis and masseter muscles with patient's teeth clenched

Ask patient to clench teeth while you palpate contracted muscles and apply opposing force. (This also tests cranial nerve V motor function.)

EXPECTED: Bilaterally symmetric with full resistance to opposition.
UNEXPECTED: Inability to produce full resistance.

CERVICAL SPINE

Inspect neck from anterior and posterior positions

- *Alignment* — **EXPECTED:** Cervical spine straight, with head erect and in approximate alignment.
- *Symmetry of skinfolds* — **UNEXPECTED:** Asymmetric skinfolds, webbed neck.

Palpate posterior neck, cervical spine, and paravertebral, trapezius, and sternocleidomastoid muscles

EXPECTED: Good muscle tone, symmetry in size.

TECHNIQUE   **FINDINGS**

UNEXPECTED: Palpable tenderness or muscle spasm.

Test range of motion

■ *Forward flexion*
Bend head forward, chin to chest.

EXPECTED: 45-degree flexion.

■ *Hyperextension*
Bend head backward, chin toward ceiling.

EXPECTED: 45-degree hyperextension.

■ *Lateral bending*
Bend head to each side, ear to each shoulder.

EXPECTED: 40-degree lateral bending.

■ *Rotation*
Turn head to each side, chin to shoulder.

EXPECTED: 70-degree rotation.

Test strength of sternocleidomastoid and trapezius muscles

Ask patient to maintain each of the previous positions while you apply opposing force. (Cranial nerve XI is also tested with rotation.)

EXPECTED: Bilaterally symmetric strength with full resistance to opposition.
UNEXPECTED: Inability to produce full resistance.

THORACIC AND LUMBAR SPINE

Inspect spine for alignment

Note major landmarks of back—each spinal process of vertebrae (C7 and T1 usually most prominent), scapulae, iliac crests, paravertebral muscles.

EXPECTED: Head positioned directly over gluteal cleft, vertebrae straight (as indicated by symmetric shoulder, scapular, and iliac crest heights), curves of cervical and lumbar spines concave, curve of thoracic spine convex, and knees and feet aligned with trunk and pointing directly forward.
UNEXPECTED: Lordosis, kyphosis, scoliosis, or sharp angular deformity (gibbus).

Palpate spinal processes and paravertebral muscles

Ask patient to stand erect.

UNEXPECTED: Muscle spasm or spinal tenderness.

TECHNIQUE	FINDINGS

Percuss for spinal tenderness

Patient is still standing erect. First, tap each spinal process with one finger, then rap each side of spine along paravertebral muscles with ulnar aspect of fist.

UNEXPECTED: Muscle spasm or spinal tenderness.

Test range of motion and curvature

Ask patient to perform following movements (mark each spinal process with skin pencil if unexpected curvature suspected):

■ *Forward flexion*
Bend forward at waist and try to touch toes. Observe patient from behind to check curvature.

EXPECTED: 75- to 90-degree flexion; back remains symmetrically flat as concave curve of lumbar spine becomes convex with forward flexion.
UNEXPECTED: Lateral curvature or rib hump.

■ *Hyperextension*
Bend back at waist as far as possible.

EXPECTED: 30-degree hypertension with reversal of lumbar curve.

■ *Lateral bending*
Bend to each side as far as possible.

EXPECTED: 35-degree lateral bending on each side.

■ *Rotation*
Swing upper trunk from waist in circular motion, front to side to back to side, while you stabilize pelvis.

EXPECTED: 30-degree rotation forward and backwad.

Test for lumbar nerve root irritation or disk herniation at L4, L5, or S1 levels (patient supine with neck slightly flexed)

■ *Straight leg raising test*
Ask patient to raise leg with knee extended. Repeat with other leg.

EXPECTED: No pain below knee with leg raising.
UNEXPECTED: Unable to raise leg more than 30 degrees without pain. Pain below knee in dermatome pattern. Flexion of knee often eliminates pain with leg raising. Crossover pain in affected leg.

TECHNIQUE	FINDINGS
■ *Bragard stretch test* Hold patient's lower leg with knee extended, and raise it slowly until pain is felt. Lower leg slightly, briskly dorsiflex foot, and internally rotate hip.	**UNEXPECTED:** Pain when leg is raised less than 70 degrees; aggravated by dorsiflexion and internal rotation of hip.

SHOULDERS

Inspect shoulders, shoulder girdle, clavicles and scapulae, area muscles

■ *Size and contour*

EXPECTED: All shoulder structures symmetric in size and contour.
UNEXPECTED: Asymmetry, hollows in rounding contour, or winged scapula.

Palpate sternoclavicular and acromioclavicular joints, clavicle, scapulae, coracoid process, greater trochanter of humerus, biceps groove, area muscles

Palpate the biceps groove by rotating the arm and forearm externally. Follow the biceps muscle and tendon along the anterior aspect of the humerus into the biceps groove.
Palpate the muscle insertion for the supraspinatus, infraspinatus, and teres minor near the greater tuberosity of the humerus by lifting the elbow posteriorly to extend the shoulder.

EXPECTED: No tenderness or masses, bilateral symmetry.
UNEXPECTED: Pain, tenderness, mass.

Test range of motion

Ask patient to perform following movements:

■ *Shoulder shrug*

EXPECTED: Symmetric rising.

■ *Forward flexion*
Raise both arms forward and straight up over head.

EXPECTED: 180-degree forward flexion.

TECHNIQUE	**FINDINGS**
■ *Hyperextension* Extend and stretch both arms behind back.	**EXPECTED:** 50-degree hyperextension.
■ *Abduction* Lift both arms laterally and straight up over head.	**EXPECTED:** 180-degree abduction.
■ *Adduction* Swing each arm across front of body.	**EXPECTED:** 50-degree adduction.
■ *Internal rotation* Place both arms behind hips, elbows out.	**EXPECTED:** 90-degree internal rotation.
■ *External rotation* Place both arms behind head, elbows out.	**EXPECTED:** 90-degree external rotation.

Test shoulder girdle muscle strength

Ask patient to maintain following positions while you apply opposing force:

■ *Shrugged shoulders*
(This also tests cranial nerve XI.)

EXPECTED: Bilaterally symmetric with full resistance to opposition.
UNEXPECTED: Inability to produce full resistance.

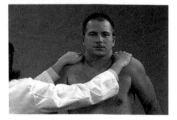

Shrugged shoulders

■ *Forward flexion*

EXPECTED: Bilaterally symmetric with full resistance to opposition.
UNEXPECTED: Inability to produce full resistance.

■ *Abduction*

EXPECTED: Bilaterally symmetric with full resistance to opposition.

TECHNIQUE	**FINDINGS**

UNEXPECTED: Inability to produce full resistance.

Assess rotator cuff muscles

Abduct the arm 90 degrees and flex the shoulders forward 30 degrees to test the supraspinatus muscle. Apply downward pressure on the distal humerus when the arm is rotated so that thumb points down or up.

UNEXPECTED: Pain and weakness with opposing force.

Flex the elbow 90 degrees and rotate the forearm medially against resistance to test the subscapularis muscle.

UNEXPECTED: Pain and weakness with opposing force.

With the arm at the side and elbow flexed 90 degrees, rotate the arm laterally against resistance to test the infraspinatus and teres minor muscles.

UNEXPECTED: Pain and weakness with opposing force.

Evaluate the rotator cuff for impingement or a tear

• *Neer test:* Have the patient internally rotate and forward flex the arm at the shoulder, pressing the supraspinatus muscle against the anterior inferior acromion.

UNEXPECTED: Increased shoulder pain.

Neer test

• *Hawkins test:* Forward flex the shoulder to 90 degrees, flexing the elbow to 90 degrees, and then internally rotating the arm to its limit.

UNEXPECTED: Increased shoulder pain.

TECHNIQUE   **FINDINGS**

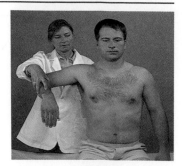

Hawkins test

ELBOWS

Inspect elbows in flexed and extended positions

- *Contour*

UNEXPECTED: Subcutaneous nodules along pressure points of extensor surface of ulna.

- *Carrying angle*
  Inspect with arms at sides passively extended, palms facing forward.

EXPECTED: Usually 5 to 15 degrees laterally.
UNEXPECTED: Lateral angle exceeding 15 degrees (cubitus valgus) or a medial carrying angle (cubitus varus).

Palpate extensor surface of ulna, olecranon process, medial and lateral epicondyles of humerus, groove on each side of olecranon process

Palpate with patient's elbow flexed at 70 degrees.

UNEXPECTED: Boggy, soft, tenderness at lateral epicondyle or along grooves of olecranon process and epicondyles.

Test range of motion

Ask patient to perform following movements:

- *Flexion and extension*
  Bend and straighten elbow.

EXPECTED: 160-degree flexion from full extension at 0 degrees.

TECHNIQUE	FINDINGS
▪ *Pronation and supination* With elbow flexed at right angle, rotate hand from palm side down to palm side up.	**EXPECTED:** 90-degree pronation and 90-degree supination. **UNEXPECTED:** Increased pain with pronation and supination of elbow.

Test muscle strength

Ask patient to maintain flexion and extension, as well as pronation and supination, while you apply opposing force.	**EXPECTED:** Bilaterally symmetric with full resistance to opposition. **UNEXPECTED:** Inability to produce full resistance.

HANDS AND WRISTS

Inspect dorsum and palm of each hand

▪ *Characteristics and contour*	**EXPECTED:** Palmar and phalangeal creases, palmar surfaces with central depression with prominent, rounded mound on thumb side (thenar eminence) and less prominent hypothenar eminence on little-finger side.
▪ *Position*	**EXPECTED:** Fingers able to fully extend and aligned with forearm when in close approximation to each other. **UNEXPECTED:** Deviation of fingers to ulnar side or inability to fully extend fingers; swan neck or boutonnière deformities.
▪ *Shape*	**EXPECTED:** Lateral finger surfaces gradually tapered from proximal to distal aspects. **UNEXPECTED:** Spindle-shaped fingers, bony overgrowths at phalangeal joints.

Palpate each joint in hand and wrist

Palpate interphalangeal joints with thumb and index finger, as	**EXPECTED:** Joint surfaces smooth.

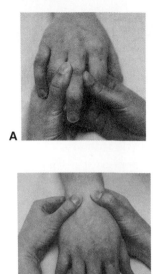

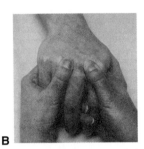

A, Palpating the interphalangeal joints with thumb and index finger.
B, Palpating metacarpophalangeal joints with both thumbs. **C,** Palpating radiocarpal groove with thumbs on dorsal surface and fingers on palmar aspect of wrist.

shown in figure above, *A;* metacarpophalangeal joints with both thumbs, as shown in figure above, *B;* and wrist and radiocarpal groove with thumbs on dorsal surface and fingers on palmar aspect of wrist, as shown in figure above, *C.*

UNEXPECTED: Nodules, swelling, bogginess, tenderness, or ganglion.

Assess integrity of median nerve

- *Tinel sign*
  Strike median nerve where it passes through carpal tunnel with index or middle finger.

UNEXPECTED: Tingling sensation radiating from wrist to hand along pathway of median nerve.

- *Thumb abduction test*
  Apply downward pressure on thumb as patient holds thumb perpendicular to hand, palm side up.

EXPECTED: Full resistance to pressure.
UNEXPECTED: Inability to produce full resistance.

TECHNIQUE	FINDINGS

■ *Phalen test*
Have patient hold both wrists in fully palmar-flexed position with dorsal surfaces pressed together for 1 minute.

UNEXPECTED: Numbness, paresthesia in distribution of median nerve.

■ *Katz hand diagram*
Have patient mark specific locations of pain, numbness, tingling in hands and arms on diagram.

UNEXPECTED: Pain, numbness, tingling in pattern shown in figure on p. 216.

Test range of motion

Ask patient to perform following movements:

■ *Metacarpophalangeal flexion and hyperextension*
Bend fingers forward at metacarpophalangeal joint, then stretch fingers up and back at knuckle.

EXPECTED: 90-degree metacarpophalangeal flexion and as much as 30-degree hyperextension.

■ *Thumb opposition*
Touch thumb to each fingertip and to base of little finger, then make a fist.

EXPECTED: Able to perform all movements.

■ *Finger abduction and adduction*
Spread fingers apart, and then touch them together.

EXPECTED: Both movements possible.

■ *Wrist extension and hyperextension*
Bend hand at wrist up and down.

EXPECTED: 90 degree flexion and 70-degree hyperextension.

■ *Radial and ulnar motion*
With palm side down, turn each hand to right and left.

EXPECTED: 20-degree radial motion and 55-degree ulnar motion.

Test muscle strength

Ask patient to perform following movements:

■ *Wrist extension and hyperextension*
Maintain wrist flexion while you apply opposing force.

EXPECTED: Bilaterally symmetric with full resistance to opposition.
UNEXPECTED: Inability to produce full resistance.

Classic pattern
Symptoms affect at least two of digits 1, 2, or 3. The classic pattern permits symptoms in the fourth and fifth digits, wrist pain, and radiation of pain proximal to the wrist, but it does not allow symptoms on the palm or dorsum of the hand.

Probable pattern
Same symptom pattern as classic except palmar symptoms are allowed unless confined solely to the ulnar aspect. In the **possible pattern,** not shown, symptoms involve only one of digits 1, 2, or 3.

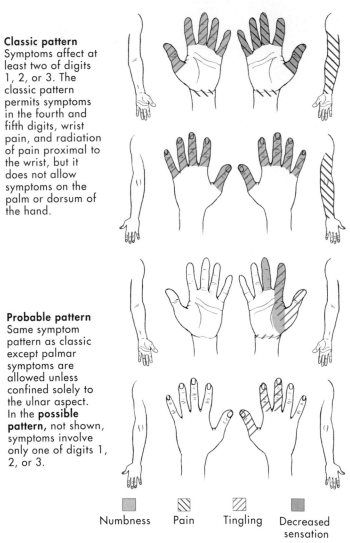

Numbness	Pain	Tingling	Decreased sensation

Redrawn from D'Arcy and McGee, 2000.

TECHNIQUE	FINDINGS

■ *Hand strength*
  Grip two of your fingers
  tightly.

EXPECTED: Firm, sustained grip.
UNEXPECTED: Weakness or pain.

HIPS

Inspect hips for symmetry and level of gluteal folds

With patient standing, inspect anteriorly and posteriorly, using major landmarks of iliac crest and greater trochanter of femur.

UNEXPECTED: Asymmetry in iliac crest height, size of buttocks, or number and level of gluteal folds.

Palpate hips and pelvis

Have patient lie supine.

UNEXPECTED: Instability, tenderness, or crepitus.

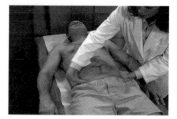

Palpating hips

Test range of motion

While in position indicated, patient should perform following movements:

■ *Flexion, knee extended*
  With patient supine, raise leg over body.

EXPECTED. Up to 90-degree flexion.

■ *Hyperextension*
  While standing or prone, swing straightened leg behind body without arching the back.

EXPECTED: Up to 30-degree hyperextension.

■ *Flexion, knee flexed*
  While supine, raise one knee to chest while keeping other leg straight.

EXPECTED: 120-degree flexion.

TECHNIQUE	FINDINGS
■ *Abduction and adduction* While supine, swing leg laterally and medially with knee straight. During adduction movement, lift patient's opposite leg to permit examined leg full movement.	**EXPECTED:** Some degree of both abduction and adduction.
■ *Internal rotation* While supine, flex knee and rotate leg inward toward other leg.	**EXPECTED:** 40-degree internal rotation.
■ *External rotation* While supine, place lateral aspect of foot on knee of other leg. Move flexed leg toward table.	**EXPECTED:** 45-degree external rotation.

Test hip muscle strength

■ *Knee in flexion and extension* Ask patient to maintain flexion of hip with knee in flexion and then extension while applying opposing force.	**EXPECTED:** Bilaterally symmetric with full resistance to opposition.
■ *Resistance to uncrossing legs while seated*	**UNEXPECTED:** Inability to produce full resistance. **EXPECTED:** Bilaterally symmetric with full resistance to opposition.

Perform Thomas test to inspect for flexion contractures

While supine, patient should fully extend one leg flat on examining table and flex other leg with knee to chest.	**EXPECTED:** Patient able to keep extended leg flat on table. **UNEXPECTED:** Extended leg lifts off table.

Thomas test

TECHNIQUE	FINDINGS

Perform Trendelenburg test to inspect for weak hip abductor muscles

Ask patient to stand and balance first on one foot, then on other. Observe from behind.

UNEXPECTED: Asymmetry or change in level of iliac crests.

LEGS AND KNEES

Inspect knees and popliteal spaces, flexed and extended

Note major landmarks—tibial tuberosity, medial and lateral tibial condyles, medial and lateral epicondyles of femur, adductor tubercle of femur, patella.

EXPECTED: Natural concavities on anterior aspect, on each side, above patella.
UNEXPECTED: Convex rather than usual concave indentation above patella.

Observe lower leg alignment

EXPECTED: Angle between femur and tibia less than 15 degrees. Bowlegs common until 18 months of age; knock knees common between 2 and 4 years.
UNEXPECTED: Knock knees (genu valgum) or bowlegs (genu varum) at other ages, excessive hyperextension of knee with weight bearing (genu recurvatum).

Palpate popliteal space

UNEXPECTED: Swelling or tenderness.

Palpate tibiofemoral joint space

Identify patella, suprapatellar pouch, infrapatellar fat pad.

EXPECTED: Smooth and firm joint.
UNEXPECTED: Tenderness, bogginess, nodules, or crepitus.

Test range of motion

■ *Flexion*
Ask patient to bend each knee.

EXPECTED: 130-degree flexion.

TECHNIQUE	**FINDINGS**
▨ *Extension* Ask patient to straighten leg and stretch it.	**EXPECTED:** Full extension and up to 15-degree hyperextension.
Test muscle strength	
▨ *Flexion and extension* Ask patient to maintain flexion and extension while you apply opposing force.	**EXPECTED:** Bilaterally symmetric with full resistance to opposition. **UNEXPECTED:** Inability to produce full resistance.

ADDITIONAL TECHNIQUES FOR KNEES

Perform ballottement procedure to determine presence of excess fluid or effusion in knee

With knee extended, apply downward pressure on suprapatellar pouch with thumb and finger of one hand, then push patella sharply downward against femur with fingers of other hand, as shown at right. Suddenly release pressure on patella, while keeping fingers lightly on knee.

UNEXPECTED: A tapping or clicking is sensed when patella is pushed against femur. Patella then floats out as if a fluid wave were pushing it.

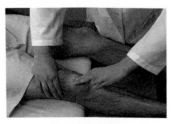

Ballottement

Test for bulge sign to determine presence of excess fluid in knee

With knee extended, milk medial aspect of knee upward two or three times, as shown in top figure on p. 221, *A*, then tap lateral side of patella, as shown in bottom figure on p. 221, *B*.

UNEXPECTED: Bulge of returning fluid to hollow area medial to patella.

TECHNIQUE   **FINDINGS**

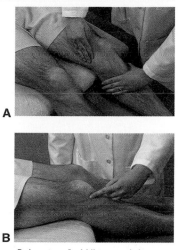

Bulge sign. **A,** Milking medial aspect of knee. **B,** Tapping patella.

Perform McMurray test to detect torn medial or lateral meniscus

Ask patient to lie supine and flex one knee completely with foot flat on table near buttocks. Maintain that flexion with your thumb and index finger on either side of the joint space while stabilizing knee. Hold heel with other hand; rotate foot and lower leg to lateral position. Extend knee to 90-degree angle. Return knee to full flexion, then repeat procedure rotating foot and lower leg to medial position.

UNEXPECTED: Palpable or audible click or limited extension of knee with either lateral or medial movements.

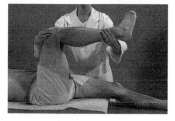

McMurray test

Perform drawer test to identify instability of anterior and posterior cruciate ligaments

Ask patient, while supine, to flex knee 45 to 90 degrees, placing foot flat on table. Place both hands on lower leg with thumbs

UNEXPECTED: Anterior or posterior movement greater than 5 mm.

TECHNIQUE	**FINDINGS**

on ridge of anterior tibia near tibial tuberosity. Pull tibia, sliding it forward of femur. Then push tibia backward.

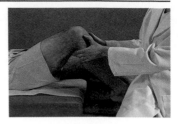

Drawer test

Perform varus and valgus stress test to identify mediolateral collateral ligament instability

Ask patient to lie supine and extend knee. While you stabilize femur with one hand and hold ankle with other, apply varus force against the ankle (toward midline) and internal rotation. Then apply valgus force against the ankle (away from midline) and external rotation. Repeat with knee flexed to 30 degrees.

UNEXPECTED: Excessive laxity felt as joint opening, medial or lateral movement.

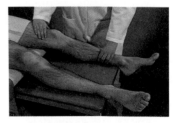

Varus and valgus stress test

Perform Apley test to detect torn meniscus

Ask patient to lie prone and flex knee to 90 degrees. Place hand on heel of foot and press firmly, opposing tibia to femur. Carefully rotate lower leg externally and internally. Do not cause excess pain.

UNEXPECTED: Clicks, locking, or pain.

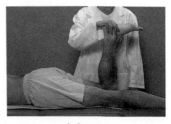

Apley test

TECHNIQUE   **FINDINGS**

FEET AND ANKLES

Inspect during weight bearing (standing and walking) and non–weight bearing

Note major landmarks—medial
malleolus, lateral malleolus,
Achilles tendon.

■ *Characteristics*   **EXPECTED:** Smooth and
                                rounded malleolar prominence,
                                prominent heels, prominent
                                metatarsophalangeal joints.
                                UNEXPECTED: Calluses and
                                corns.

■ *Alignment*   **EXPECTED:** Feet aligned with
                                tibias and weight bearing on foot
                                midline.
                                UNEXPECTED: In-toeing
                                (pes varus), out-toeing (pes
                                valgus), deviations in forefoot
                                alignment (metatarsus varus or
                                metatarsus valgus), heel
                                pronation, or pain.

■ *Contour*   **EXPECTED:** Longitudinal
                                arch that may flatten with weight
                                bearing. Foot flat when not
                                bearing weight (pes planus) and
                                high instep (pes cavus) are
                                common variations.
                                UNEXPECTED: Pain with
                                pes planus.

■ *Toes*   **EXPECTED:** Toes on each
                                foot straight forward, flat, in
                                alignment.
                                UNEXPECTED: Hammertoe;
                                claw toe; mallet toe; hallux
                                valgus; bunions; or heat, redness,
                                swelling, tenderness of metatarso-
                                phalangeal joint of great toe
                                (possibly with draining tophus).

Palpate Achilles tendon and each metatarsal joint

Using thumb and fingers of both   **EXPECTED:** No tenderness or
hands, compress forefoot, palpating   masses, bilateral symmetry.

TECHNIQUE	FINDINGS
each metatarsophalangeal joint.	**UNEXPECTED:** Pain, masses, thickened Achilles tendon.

Test range of motion

Ask patient to sit, then perform following movements:

- ▪ *Dorsiflexion*
  Point foot toward ceiling.

EXPECTED: 20-degree dorsiflexion.

- ▪ *Plantar flexion*
  Point foot toward floor.

EXPECTED: 45-degree plantar flexion.

- ▪ *Inversion and eversion*
  Bend foot at ankle, then turn sole of foot toward and away from other foot.

EXPECTED: 30-degree inversion and 20-degree eversion.

- ▪ *Abduction and adduction*
  Rotate ankle, turning away from and then toward other foot (while you stabilize leg).

EXPECTED: 10-degree abduction and 20-degree adduction.

- ▪ *Flexion and extension*
  Bend and straighten toes.

EXPECTED: Some flexion and extension, especially of great toes.

Test strength of ankle muscles

Ask patient to maintain dorsiflexion and plantar flexion while you apply opposing force.

EXPECTED: Bilaterally symmetric with full resistance to opposition.
UNEXPECTED: Inability to produce full resistance.

AIDS TO DIFFERENTIAL DIAGNOSIS

ABNORMALITY	DESCRIPTION
Carpal tunnel syndrome	Numbness, burning, tingling in hands, often occurring at night but also elicited by rotational movement of wrist. Pain in arms. Can result in weakness of hand and flattening of thenar eminence of palm.
Gout	Red, hot, swollen joint (classically proximal phalanx of great toe, although other joints of wrist, hands, ankles, knees are sometimes affected); exquisite

ABNORMALITY	DESCRIPTION
	pain; limited range of motion; tophi; and mild fever. Skin over joint may be shiny and red or purple.
Lumbar disk herniation	Lower back pain with radiation to buttocks and posterior thigh or down leg in distribution of nerve root dermatome (see pp. 237-238), spasm or tenderness over paraspinal muscles, muscle weakness, paresthesia. Numbness, tingling, or weakness of involved extremity.
Bursitis	Motion limitation caused by swelling, pain on movement, point tenderness, erythema, warmth; commonly occurs in shoulder, elbow, hip, knee.
Osteoarthritis	See table on p. 226.
Rheumatoid arthritis	See table on p. 226.
Sprain	Pain, marked swelling, hemorrhage, loss of function associated with stretching or tearing of a joint ligament.
Fracture	Deformity, edema, pain, loss of function, color changes, paresthesia associated with break or crush injury to a bone.
Tenosynovitis (tendinitis)	Point tenderness over involved tendon; edema; pain with active movement; and some limitation of movement in affected joint.
Rotator cuff tear	Severe pain in shoulder, deltoid area, over acromioclavicular joint; inability to abduct arm or maintain arm in abduction due to pain, inability to shrug shoulders, weakness in external shoulder rotation; grating sound on movement, crepitus.
Scoliosis	Uneven shoulder and hip levels, rib hump, flank asymmetry on forward flexion. Lateral curvature of spine resulting from

ABNORMALITY	DESCRIPTION
	leg length discrepancy also possible (functional scoliosis).
Osteoporosis	Height loss, bent spine, appearance of sinking into hips—most often in postmenopausal women and some persons on corticosteroids for disease management. Usual presenting symptom is acute, painful fracture, most commonly of hip, vertebra, or wrist.

Differential Diagnosis of Arthritis

Signs and Symptoms	Osteoarthritis	Rheumatoid Arthritis
Onset	Insidious	Gradual or sudden (24-48 hours)
Duration of stiffness	Few minutes, localized, but short "gelling" after prolonged rest	Often hours, most pronounced after rest
Pain	On motion, with prolonged activity, relieved by rest	Even at rest, may disturb sleep
Weakness	Usually localized and not severe	Often pronounced, out of proportion with muscle atrophy
Fatigue	Unusual	Often severe, with onset 4 to 5 hours after rising
Emotional depression and lability	Unusual	Common, coincides with fatigue and disease activity, often relieved if in remission
Tenderness over localized afflicted joint	Common	Almost always; most sensitive indicator of inflammation
Swelling	Effusion common, little synovial, reaction swelling rare	Fusiform soft tissue enlargement, effusion common, synovial proliferation and thickening
Heat, erythema	Unusual	Sometimes present
Crepitus, crackling	Coarse to medium on motion	Medium to fine
Joint enlargement	Mild with firm consistency	Moderate to severe

Modified from McCarty, 1993.

PEDIATRIC VARIATIONS

EXAMINATION

Musculoskeletal findings and motor development in infants, children, and adolescents change as they grow. For a complete description of age-specific anticipated pediatric findings, see Chapter 21.

SPORTS PARTICIPATION SCREENING EXAMINATION FOR CHILDREN AND ADOLESCENTS

- Observe posture and general muscle contour bilaterally.
- Observe gait.
- Ask patient to walk on tiptoes and heels.
- Observe patient hop on each foot.
- Ask patient to duck walk four steps with knees completely bent.
- Inspect spine for curvature and lumbar extension, fingers touching toes with knees straight.
- Palpate shoulder and clavicle for dislocation.
- Check following for range of motion—neck, shoulder, elbow, forearm, hands, fingers, hips.
- Test knee ligaments for drawer sign.

SAMPLE DOCUMENTATION

Subjective. A 13-year-old female referred by school nurse because of uneven shoulder and hip heights. Active in sports, good strength, no back pain or stiffness.

Objective. Spine straight without obvious deformities when erect, but mild right curvature of thoracic spine with forward flexion. No rib hump. Right shoulder and iliac crest slightly higher than left. Muscles and extremities symmetric; muscle strength appropriate and equal bilaterally; active range of motion without pain, locking, clicking, or limitation in all joints.

NEUROLOGIC SYSTEM

EQUIPMENT

- Familiar objects (coins, keys, paper clip)
- Vials of aromatic substances (coffee, orange, peppermint, banana)
- Sterile needles
- Cotton wisp
- Tongue blades (one intact and one broken with pointed and rounded edges)
- List of tastes
- Vials of solutions (glucose, salt, lemon or vinegar, quinine) with applicators
- Cup of water
- Test tubes of hot and cold water
- Tuning forks
- Reflex hammer
- 5.07 monofilament

EXAMINATION

Evaluate the neurologic system as the rest of the body is examined. When history and examination findings have not revealed a potential neurologic problem, perform a neurologic screening examination as shown in the box on p. 229, rather than a full neurologic examination. See Chapter 17, Musculoskeletal System, for evaluation of muscle tone and strength, as these findings are important for interpreting neurologic system examination findings. The mental status portion of the neurologic system examination is found in Chapter 2.

Neurologic Screening Examination

This shorter screening examination is commonly used for health visits when no known neurologic problem is apparent.

Cranial Nerves
Cranial nerves II through XII are routinely tested; however, taste and smell are not tested unless some aberration is found.

Proprioception and Cerebellar Function
One test is administered for each of the following: rapid rhythmic alternating movements, accuracy of movements, balance (Romberg test), gait, and heel-toe walking.

Sensory Function
Superficial pain and touch at a distal point in each extremity are tested; vibration and position senses are assessed by testing the great toe.

Deep Tendon Reflexes
All deep tendon reflexes and the plantar reflex are tested, excluding the test for clonus.

CRANIAL NERVES I-XII

The table below summarizes the cranial nerve (CN) examination. When a sensory or motor loss is suspected, be compulsive about determining the extent of the loss.

Procedures for Cranial Nerve Examination

Cranial Nerve (CN)	Procedure
CN I (olfactory)	Test ability to identify familiar aromatic odors, one naris at a time with eyes closed.
CN II (optic)	Test vision with Snellen chart and Rosenbaum near-vision chart.
	Perform ophthalmoscopic examination of fundi.
	Test visual fields by confrontation and extinction of vision.
CN III, CN IV, CN VI (oculomotor, trochlear, abducens)	Test extraocular movement.
	Inspect eyelids for drooping
	Inspect pupil size for equality and direct and consensual response to light and accommodation.

Continued

Procedures for Cranial Nerve Examination—cont'd

Cranial Nerve (CN)	Procedure
CN V (trigeminal)	Inspect face for muscle atrophy and tremors. Palpate jaw muscles for tone and strength when patient clenches teeth. Test superficial pain and touch sensation in each branch. (Test temperature sensation if there are unexpected findings to pain or touch.) Test corneal reflex.
CN VII (facial)	Inspect symmetry of facial features with various expressions (e.g., smile, frown, puffed cheeks, wrinkled forehead). Test ability to identify sweet and salty tastes on each side of tongue.
CN VIII (acoustic)	Test sense of hearing with whisper screening tests or by audiometry. Compare bone and air conduction of sound. Test for lateralization of sound.
CN IX (glossopharyngeal)	Test ability to identify sour and bitter tastes. Test gag reflex and ability to swallow.
CN X (vagus)	Inspect palate and uvula for symmetry with speech sounds and gag reflex. Observe for swallowing difficulty. Evaluate quality of guttural speech sounds (presence of nasal or hoarse quality to voice).
CN XI (spinal accessory)	Test trapezius muscle strength (shrug shoulders against resistance). Test sternocleidomastoid muscle strength (turn head to each side against resistance).
CN XII (hypoglossal)	Inspect tongue in mouth and while protruded for symmetry, tremors, atrophy. Inspect tongue movement toward nose and chin. Test tongue strength with index finger when tongue is pressed against cheek. Evaluate quality of lingual speech sounds (l, t, d, n).

TECHNIQUE

FINDINGS

Assess olfactory nerve (CN I)

Ask patient to close eyes. Occlude one naris, hold vial (using least irritating aromatic substances first [e.g., orange or peppermint extract]) under nose, and ask patient to breathe deeply and identify odor. Allow patient to

EXPECTED: Able to perceive and usually identify odor on each side.

UNEXPECTED: Anosmia, loss of smell or inability to discriminate odors.

TECHNIQUE	**FINDINGS**

breathe comfortably, then occlude
other naris and repeat with different
odor. Continue, alternating two
or three odors.

Assess optic nerve (CN II)

See tests for visual acuity and
visual fields in Chapter 7, Eyes.

Assess oculomotor, trochlear, abducens nerves (CN III, CN IV, CN VI)

See tests for six cardinal points of
gaze, pupil size, shape, response
to light and accommodation, and
opening of upper eyelids in
Chapter 7, Eyes.

EXPECTED: Equal pupil size,
equal and consensual response
to light and accommodation,
symmetric eye movements in
all six cardinal points of gaze.
UNEXPECTED: Absence of
lateral gaze. Absence of any
expected findings, ptosis.

Assess trigeminal nerve (CN V)

■ *Facial muscle tone*
Ask patient to clench teeth
tightly as you palpate muscles
over jaw.

■ *Sensation*
Ask patient to close eyes and
report if sensation to touch is
present or is sharp or dull as
you touch each side of face at
scalp, cheek, and chin areas,
alternately using sharp and
rounded edges of tongue blade
or paper clip in an unpredictable
pattern. Ask patient to report
when the stimulus is felt as
you stroke same six areas with
cotton wisp or brush. Finally,
test sensation over buccal
mucosa with wooden applicator.

■ *Corneal reflex*
See test for corneal sensitivity in
Chapter 7, Eyes.

EXPECTED: Symmetric tone.
UNEXPECTED: Muscle
atrophy, deviation of jaw to one
side, or fasciculations.
EXPECTED: Symmetric
discrimination of sensations in
each location to all stimuli.
UNEXPECTED: Impaired
sensation. If impaired, use test
tubes of hot and cold water to
evaluate temperature sensation.

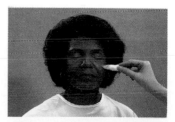

Testing sensation over distribution
of cranial nerve V.

TECHNIQUE	**FINDINGS**

Assess facial nerve (CN VII)

■ *Expressions*
Assess motor function by asking patient to make the following facial expressions:
Raise eyebrows and wrinkle forehead
Smile
Frown
Puff out cheeks
Purse lips and blow out
Show teeth
Squeeze eyes shut against resistance

EXPECTED: Facial symmetry.
UNEXPECTED: Tics, unusual facial movements, or asymmetry of expression (flattened nasolabial fold, lower eyelid sagging, side of mouth drooping).

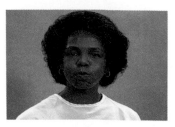

Assessing motor function of cranial nerve VII.

■ *Speech*
Listen to articulation and clarity of speech
■ *Taste (CN VII and CN IX)*
Hold card listing tastes in patient's view. Ask patient to extend tongue. Apply one of four solutions to lateral side of tongue in appropriate tastebud region. Ask patient to point to taste perceived. Offer patient a sip of water, and repeat with different solution and applicator, testing each side of tongue with each solution,

UNEXPECTED: Difficulties with enunciating *b, m,* and *p* (labial sounds).
EXPECTED: Able to identify sweet, salty, sour, bitter taste bilaterally when placed in appropriate tastebud region.

Assess acoustic nerve (CN VIII)

■ *Hearing*
See screening tests in Chapter 8, Ears, Nose, and Throat, or use an audiometer to test hearing.
■ *Balance*
See Romberg test, p. 235.

EXPECTED: Adequate hearing bilaterally.

TECHNIQUE	FINDINGS

Assess glossopharyngeal nerve (CN IX)

▧ *Taste*
See CN VII.

▧ *Gag reflex (nasopharyngeal sensation)*
See CN X.

Assess vagus nerve (CN X)

▧ *Gag reflex (nasopharyngeal sensation) (CN IX and CN X)*
Tell patient you will be testing gag reflex. Touch posterior wall of pharynx with applicator while observing palate, pharyngeal muscles, and uvula.

EXPECTED: Upward movement of palate and contraction of pharyngeal muscles, with uvula in midline.
UNEXPECTED: Drooping or absence of arch on either side of soft palate; uvula deviates from midline.

▧ *Motor function*
Ask patient to say "ah" while observing movement of soft palate and uvula.

UNEXPECTED: Failure of soft palate to rise or deviation of uvula from midline.

▧ *Swallowing (CN IX and CN X)*
Ask patient to swallow water.

EXPECTED: Water easily swallowed.
UNEXPECTED: Retrograde passage of water through nose

▧ *Speech*

UNEXPECTED: Hoarseness, nasal quality, or difficulty with guttural sounds.

Assess spinal accessory nerve (CN XI)

See Chapter 6, Head and Neck, and Chapter 17, Musculoskeletal System, for evaluations of size, shape, strength of trapezius and sternocleidomastoid muscles.

EXPECTED: Symmetric size, shape, and strength.

Assess hypoglossal nerve (CN XII)

▧ *Tongue resting and protruded*
Inspect while at rest on floor of mouth and while protruded.

EXPECTED: Tongue midline, symmetric size.
UNEXPECTED: Fasciculations, asymmetry, atrophy, or deviation from midline.

TECHNIQUE   **FINDINGS**

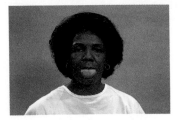

Assessing motor function of cranial
nerve XII.

■ *Tongue movement*
Ask patient to move tongue in
and out, side to side, curled up
toward nose, curled down
toward chin.

EXPECTED: Able to perform
most tongue movements.

■ *Tongue strength*
Ask patient to push tongue
against cheek while you apply
resistance with index finger.

EXPECTED: Steady, firm
pressure.

■ *Speech*

UNEXPECTED: Problems
with *l, t, d,* or *n* (lingual sounds).

PROPRIOCEPTION AND CEREBELLAR FUNCTION

Evaluate coordination and fine motor skills

Have patient sit.

■ *Rapid, rhythmic, alternating
movements*
Ask patient to pat knees with
both hands, alternately patting
with palmar and dorsal surfaces
of the hands. Alternatively, ask
the patient to touch the
thumb to each finger
of the same hand sequentially
from index finger to little finger
and back, one hand at a time.

EXPECTED: Smooth
execution, maintaining rhythm
with increasing speed.
UNEXPECTED: Stiff, slowed,
nonrhythmic, or jerky clonic
movements.

■ *Accuracy of movement: Finger-
to-finger test*
Position your index finger 40
to 50 cm from patient. Ask
patient to alternately touch his
or her nose and your index

EXPECTED: Movements
rapid, smooth, accurate.
UNEXPECTED: Consistent
past pointing (missing
examiner's index finger).

TECHNIQUE	**FINDINGS**

finger with the index finger of one hand, as shown below. Change location of your index finger several times. Repeat with patient's other hand.

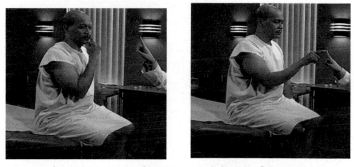

Assessing accuracy of movement with finger-to-finger test.

■ *Accuracy of movement: Finger-to-nose test*
Ask patient to close both eyes and touch his or her nose with index finger of each hand while alternating hands and gradually increasing speed.

EXPECTED: Movements rapid, smooth, accurate, even with increasing speed.

■ *Accuracy of movement: Heel-to-shin test* (can be performed sitting, standing, or supine). Ask patient to run heel of one foot along shin of opposite leg from knee to ankle. Repeat with other heel.

EXPECTED: Able to move heel up and down shin in straight line.
UNEXPECTED: Irregular deviations to side.

Evaluate balance

■ *Balance: Romberg test*
Ask patient to stand with feet together and arms at sides, with eyes first open, then closed. **Stand close by in case patient starts to fall.**

EXPECTED: Slight swaying movement, no danger of falling.
UNEXPECTED: Staggering, losing balance, or swaying to the extent of falling.

■ *Balance: Recovery*
After explaining test to patient, ask patient to spread feet slightly, then push shoulders to

EXPECTED: Quick recovery of balance.
UNEXPECTED: Must catch patient to prevent a fall.

TECHNIQUE	FINDINGS

throw patient off balance.
Be prepared to catch patient.

- *Balance: Standing and hopping*
Have patient stand in place on one foot, then the other, with eyes open. Then have patient hop on each foot.

EXPECTED: Able to stand and hop 5 seconds on each foot without losing balance.
UNEXPECTED: Instability, need to continually touch floor with opposite foot, or tendency to fall.

- *Gait: Walking*
Ask patient to walk without shoes around examining room or down hallway, with eyes first open, then closed.

EXPECTED: Smooth, regular gait rhythm and symmetric stride length; upright trunk posture swaying with gait phase; and arm swing smooth and symmetric.
UNEXPECTED: Shuffling, widely placed feet, toe walking, foot flop, leg lag, scissoring, loss of arm swing, staggering, lurching, or waddling motion.

- *Gait: Heel-toe walking*
Ask patient to walk a straight line, first forward and then backward, with eyes open and arms at side. Ask patient to touch toe of one foot with heel of other.

EXPECTED: Consistent contact between toe and heel with slight swaying.
UNEXPECTED: Extension of arms for balance, instability, tendency to fall, or lateral staggering and reeling.

SENSORY FUNCTION

Test primary sensory functions

Ask patient to close eyes for all tests. Use minimal stimulation initially, then increase gradually until patient becomes aware. Test contralateral areas, asking patient to compare perceived sensations side to side.

EXPECTED: For all tests, minimal differences side to side, correct interpretation of sensations, discrimination of side of body tested, location of sensation (e.g., proximal or distal to previous stimulus).
UNEXPECTED: For all tests, map boundaries of any impairment by distribution of major peripheral nerves or dermatomes (see figures on pp. 237-238).

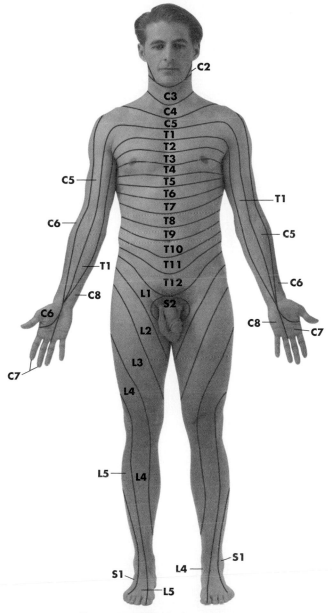

Dermatomes of the body, anterior view

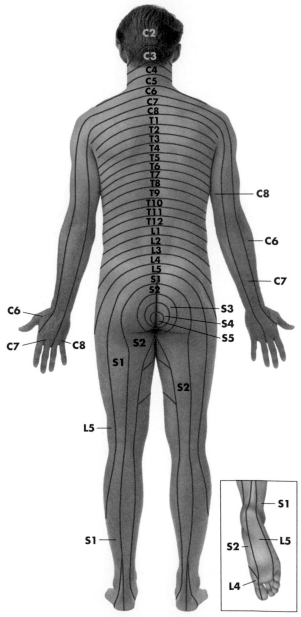

Dermatomes of the body, posterior view

TECHNIQUE	FINDINGS

■ *Superficial touch*
Lightly touch skin with cotton wisp or your fingertips, as shown at right. Ask patient to point to area touched or acknowledge when sensation is felt.

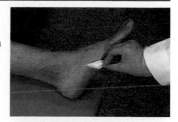

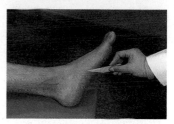

Superficial touch assessment

■ *Superficial pain*
Alternating sharp and smooth edges of broken tongue blade or point and hub of sterile needle or paperclip, touch skin in unpredictable pattern. Ask patient to identify sensation (sharp or dull) and where it is felt.

■ *Temperature and deep pressure*
Perform test only if superficial pain sensation is not intact.
Temperature: Alternately roll test tubes of hot and cold water against skin in an unpredictable pattern. Ask patient to indicate hot or cold and where it is felt.
Deep pressure: Squeeze trapezius, calf, or biceps muscle.

EXPECTED: Discomfort with deep pressure.

TECHNIQUE	FINDINGS

- *Protective sensation*
  Perform test only if patient has diabetes mellitus or peripheral neuropathy. Apply 5.07 monofilament until filament bends. Use a random pattern to test several sites on plantar surface of foot and once on dorsal surface. Avoid calloused areas and broken skin.

EXPECTED: Sensation felt at all sites touched.
UNEXPECTED: Loss of sensation at any site.

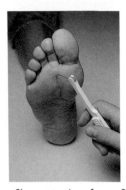

Monofilament testing of superficial touch

- *Vibration*
  Place stem of vibrating tuning fork against several bony prominences (e.g., toes, ankle, shin, finger joints, wrist, elbow, shoulder, sternum), beginning distally. Ask patient when and where sensation is felt and what it feels like. Dampen tines occasionally to see whether patient notices the difference.

EXPECTED: Buzzing or tingling sensation.
UNEXPECTED: Does not distinguish vibration from touch of tuning fork.

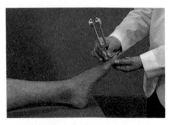

Assessment of vibration sensation

- *Position of joints*
  Hold joint to be tested (great toe or finger) by lateral aspects in neutral position, then raise or lower digit, as shown, and

EXPECTED: Patient correctly identifies position of joint.

TECHNIQUE	FINDINGS

ask patient which way it was moved. Return to neutral before moving in another direction. Repeat so both feet and both hands are tested.

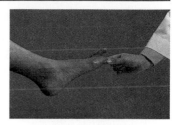

Position sense assessment

Test cortical sensory functions

Ask patient to close eyes for all tests.

■ *Stereognosis*
Hand patient familiar objects (e.g., key, coin), and ask patient to identify.

UNEXPECTED: Inability to recognize objects (tactile agnosia).

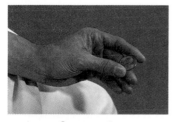

Stereognosis

■ *Two-point discrimination*
Using two sterile needles or paper-clip ends, alternately touch patient's skin with one or both points simultaneously at various locations. Find distance at which patient can no longer distinguish two points.

EXPECTED: See table on p. 242.

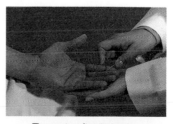

Two-point discrimination

■ *Extinction phenomenon*
Simultaneously touch cheek and hand, or two other areas

EXPECTED: Location of both sensations identified.

Minimal Distances of Discriminating Two Points

Body Part	Minimal Distance (mm)
Tongue	1
Fingertips	2-8
Toes	3-8
Palms of hands	8-12
Chest and forearms	40
Back	40-70
Upper arms and thighs	75

From Barkauskas et al, 2001.

TECHNIQUE	FINDINGS

on each side of body with sterile needles. Ask patient the number of stimuli and locations.

■ *Graphesthesia*
With blunt pen or applicator stick, draw letter or number on palm of patient's hand, and ask patient to identify it. Repeat with different figure on other hand.

EXPECTED: Letter or number readily recognized.

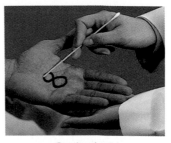

Graphesthesia

■ *Point location*
Touch area on patient's skin and withdraw stimulus. Ask patient to point to area touched.

EXPECTED: Able to locate stimulus.

REFLEXES

Test superficial reflexes

Have patient supine.
■ *Abdominal*
Stroke each quadrant of abdomen with end of reflex

EXPECTED: Slight, bilaterally equal movement of umbilicus toward each area of stimulation.

TECHNIQUE   **FINDINGS**

hammer or with tongue
blade edge.

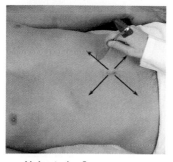

Abdominal reflex assessment

■ *Cremasteric (male patients)*   **EXPECTED:** Testicle and
Stroke inner thigh, proximal   scrotum rise on stroked side.
to distal.
■ *Plantar reflex*   **EXPECTED:** Plantar flexion
Using pointed object, stroke   of all toes.
lateral side of foot from heel   **UNEXPECTED:** Fanning of
to ball, then curve across ball   toes or dorsiflexion of great toe
to medial side.   with or without fanning of
                                        other toes (Babinski sign—
                                        expected in children under
                                        2 years).

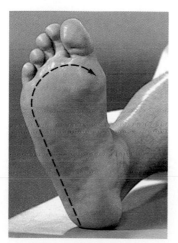

Plantar reflex assessment

TECHNIQUE	**FINDINGS**

Test deep tendon reflexes

Patient relaxed and either sitting or lying for most procedures. Test each reflex, comparing responses on corresponding sides. Score deep tendon reflexes on scale shown in table below.

EXPECTED: Symmetric visible or palpable responses. **UNEXPECTED:** Absent or diminished responses (0 or 1 +), or hyperactive reflexes (3 + or 4 +).

Scoring Deep Tendon Reflexes

Grade	Deep Tendon Reflex Response
0	No response
1 +	Sluggish or diminished
2 +	Active or expected response
3 +	More brisk than expected, slightly hyperactive
4 +	Brisk, hyperactive, with intermittent or transient clonus

■ *Biceps*
Flex arm 45 degrees at elbow, then palpate biceps tendon in antecubital fossa. Place thumb over tendon and fingers under elbow. Strike your thumb with reflex hammer.

EXPECTED: Visible or palpable flexion of elbow, contraction of biceps muscle.

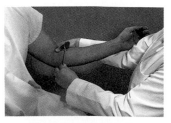

Biceps deep tendon reflex

■ *Brachioradial*
Flex patient's arm up to 45 degrees while resting patient's forearm on your arm, with hand slightly pronated. Strike brachioradial tendon.

EXPECTED: Pronation of forearm and flexion of elbow.

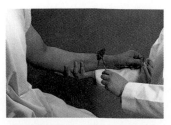

Brachioradialis deep tendon reflex

TECHNIQUE	**FINDINGS**

■ *Triceps*
Flex patient's arm at elbow up to 90 degrees and allow patient's lower arm to hang freely, or rest patient's forearm on your arm. Palpate triceps tendon and strike directly with reflex hammer, just above elbow.

EXPECTED: Visible or palpable extension of elbow, contraction of triceps muscle.

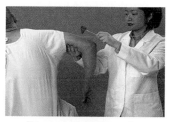

Triceps deep tendon reflex

■ *Patellar*
Flex patient's knee up to 90 degrees, allowing lower leg to hang loosely. Support upper leg so it does not rest against edge of examining table, then strike patellar tendon just below patella.

EXPECTED: Extension of lower leg, contraction of quadriceps muscle.

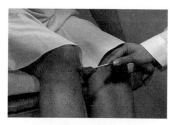

Patellar deep tendon reflex

■ *Achilles*
Ask patient to sit. Then flex patient's knee and dorsiflex ankle up to 90 degrees, holding heel of foot. Strike Achilles tendon at level of ankle malleoli.

EXPECTED: Plantar flexion, contraction of gastrocnemius muscle.

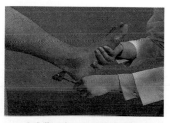

Achilles deep tendon reflex

■ *Clonus*
Support patient's knee in

UNEXPECTED: Sustained clonus, rhythmic oscillating

TECHNIQUE	FINDINGS
partially flexed position and briskly dorsiflex foot with other hand, maintaining foot in flexion.	movements between dorsiflexion and plantar flexion palpated.

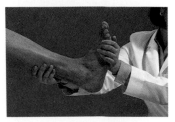

Clonus assessment

Differential Diagnosis of Upper and Lower Motor Neuron Disorders

Assessment Parameters	Upper Motor Neuron	Lower Motor Neuron
Muscle tone	Increased tone, muscle spasticity, risk for contractures	Decreased tone, muscle flaccidity
Muscle atrophy	Little or no muscle atrophy, but decreased strength	Loss of muscle strength; muscle atrophy or wasting
Sensation	Sensation loss may affect entire limb	Sensory loss following distribution of dermatomes or peripheral nerves
Reflexes	Hyperactive deep tendon and abdominal reflexes; positive Babinski sign	Weak or absent deep tendon, plantar, and abdominal reflexes, absent Babinski sign, no pathologic reflexes
Fasciculation	No fasciculations	Fasciculations
Motor effect	Paralysis of voluntary movements	Paralysis of muscles
Location of insult	Damage above level of brainstem will affect contralateral side of body, damage below the brainstem will affect the ipsilateral side of the body	Damage affects muscle on ipsilateral side of body

AIDS TO DIFFERENTIAL DIAGNOSIS

ABNORMALITY	DESCRIPTION
Generalized seizure disorder	Episodic, sudden, involuntary contractions of a group of muscles resulting from excessive discharge of cerebral neurons. Disturbances in conscious behavior, sensation, autonomic functioning, urinary and fecal incontinence may accompany seizures.
Meningitis	Inflammatory process of meninges. Fever, chills, nuchal rigidity, headache, seizures, vomiting, followed by alterations in level of consciousness. ***Can be life-threatening.***
Encephalitis	Inflammation of brain and spinal cord that often begins as a mild, febrile viral illness, often followed by a quiescent stage. Headache, drowsiness, confusion, lethargy, and coma. Possible motor function impairment and muscle weakness with severe paralysis or ataxia.
Lesions (intracranial)	Headaches, vomiting, change in cognition, motor dysfunction, unsteady gait, papilledema, seizures, behavioral or personality changes.
Cerebrovascular accident (brain attack or stroke)	Sudden, focal neurologic deficit resulting from impaired circulation of brain. Sudden weakness, numbness or paralysis of face, arms, or legs, often unilateral. Sudden trouble seeing in one or both eyes. Sudden confusion, difficulty speaking or understanding speech. Sudden severe headache. Sudden trouble walking, loss of balance, or loss of coordination.

ABNORMALITY	DESCRIPTION
Parkinson disease	Initial symptoms: Tremors at rest and with fatigue that disappear with intended movement and sleep. Progressive symptoms: tremor of head; slowing of voluntary movement; bilateral pill-rolling of fingers; delays in execution of movement; masked facial expression; poor blink rate; short, shuffling steps; slowed, slurred, monotonous speech; and possible behavioral changes and dementia. Late symptoms: postural instability.
Peripheral neuropathy	Decreased or loss of pain, vibratory, temperature sensation; absent reflexes and muscle wasting in affected extremity sometimes occurs. Most common in hands and feet.
Cerebral palsy	Alterations in muscle tone, posture, motor performance, reflexes, sensory impairment.

PEDIATRIC VARIATIONS

EXAMINATION

Neurologic findings in the infant and child change as the child matures. For a complete description of anticipated maturational findings see Chapter 21.

TECHNIQUE	FINDINGS
Indirectly evaluate cranial nerves in newborns and infants	
■ *Optical blink reflex (CN II, CN III, CN IV, CN VI)* Shine a light at infant's open eyes. Observe quick closure of eyes and dorsal flexion of head.	**EXPECTED:** Gazes intensely at close object or face. Focuses on and tracks an object with both eyes. **UNEXPECTED:** No response may indicate poor light perception.

TECHNIQUE	FINDINGS
■ *Rooting reflex (CN V)* Touch one corner of infant's mouth.	**EXPECTED:** Infant should open mouth and turn head in direction of stimulation. If infant has been fed recently, minimal or no response is expected.
■ *Sucking reflex (CN V)* Place your finger in infant's mouth, feeling sucking action. Note pressure, strength, pattern of sucking.	**EXPECTED:** Tongue should push up against your finger with good strength.
■ *Infant's facial expression (CN VII)* Observe and note infant's ability to wrinkle forehead when crying and symmetry of smile.	**EXPECTED:** Facial symmetry with all expressions.
■ *Acoustic blink reflex (CN VIII)* Loudly clap your hands about 30 cm from infant's head; avoid producing an air current.	**EXPECTED:** Blink in response to sound. Infant will habituate to repeated testing. Freezes position with high-pitched sound. **UNEXPECTED:** No response after 2 to 3 days of age may indicate hearing problems.
■ *Doll's eye maneuver (CN VIII)* Hold infant under axilla in upright position, head held steady, facing you. Rotate infant first in one direction and then in other.	**EXPECTED:** Infant's eyes should turn in direction of rotation and then opposite direction when rotation stops. **UNEXPECTED:** If eyes do not move in expected direction, suspect vestibular problem or eye muscle paralysis.
■ *Swallowing and gag reflex (CN IX and CN X)* ■ *Sucking and swallowing (CN XII)* Pinch infant's nose.	**EXPECTED:** Coordinated sucking and swallowing ability. Mouth will open, and tip of tongue will rise in midline position.

TECHNIQUE	FINDINGS

Evaluate primitive reflexes in infant

■ *Palmar grasp (present at birth)* Making sure infant's head is in midline, touch palm of infant's hand from ulnar side (opposite thumb).

EXPECTED: Strong grasp of your finger. Sucking facilitates grasp. Grasp should be strongest between 1 and 2 months of age and disappear by 3 month

■ *Plantar grasp (present at birth)* Touch plantar surface of infant's feet at the base of toes.

EXPECTED: Toes should curl downward. Reflex should be strong up to 8 months of age.

■ *Moro reflex (present at birth)* With infant supported in semisitting position, allow head and trunk to drop back to a 30-degree angle.

EXPECTED: Symmetric abduction and extension of arms. Fingers fan out, and thumb and index finger form a "c." Arms then adduct in an embracing motion followed by relaxed flexion. Reflex diminishes in strength by 3 to 4 months and disappears by 6 months.

■ *Placing (4 days of age)* Hold infant upright under axilla next to a table or chair. Touch dorsal side of foot to table or chair edge.

EXPECTED: Flexion of hips and knees and lifting of foot as if stepping up on table. Age of disappearance varies.

■ *Stepping (between birth and 8 weeks)* Hold infant upright under axilla and allow soles of feet to touch surface of table.

EXPECTED: Alternate flexion and extension of legs, simulating walking. Disappears before voluntary walking.

■ *Asymmetric tonic neck or "fencing" (by 2 to 3 months)* With infant lying supine and relaxed or sleeping, turn infant's head to one side so jaw is over shoulder.

EXPECTED: Extension of arm and leg on side to which head is turned and flexion of opposite arm and leg.

Turn infant's head to other side

EXPECTED: Reversal of extremities' posture. Reflex diminishes at 3 to 4 months of age and disappears by 6 months.

TECHNIQUE	FINDINGS
	UNEXPECTED: Be concerned if infant never exhibits reflex or seems locked in fencing position.

Evaluate neurologic soft signs in children

Age at which finding becomes unexpected noted in parentheses.

TECHNIQUE	FINDINGS
■ *Walking, running gait*	**UNEXPECTED:** Stiff-legged with foot-slapping quality, unusual posturing of arm (3 years).
■ *Heel walking*	**UNEXPECTED:** Difficulty remaining on heels for distance of 10 feet (7 years).
■ *Tiptoe walking*	**UNEXPECTED:** Difficulty remaining on toes for distance of 10 feet (7 years).
■ *Tandem gait*	**UNEXPECTED:** Difficulty walking heel to toe, unusual posturing of arms (7 years).
■ *One-foot standing*	**UNEXPECTED:** Unable to remain standing on one foot longer than 5 to 10 seconds (5 years).
■ *Hopping in place*	**UNEXPECTED:** Unable to rhythmically hop on each foot (6 years).
■ *Motor stance*	**UNEXPECTED:** Difficulty maintaining stance (arms extended in front, feet together, eyes closed), drifting of arms, mild writhing movements of hands or fingers (3 years).
■ *Visual tracking*	**UNEXPECTED:** Difficulty following object with eyes when keeping head still; nystagmus (5 years).

TECHNIQUE	FINDINGS
Rapid thumb-to-finger test	**UNEXPECTED:** Rapid touching of thumb to fingers in sequence is uncoordinated; unable to suppress mirror movements in contralateral hand (8 years).
Rapid alternating movements of hands	**UNEXPECTED:** Irregular speed and rhythm with pronation and supination of hands patting knees (10 years).
Finger-nose test	**UNEXPECTED:** Unable to alternately touch examiner's finger and own nose consecutively (7 years).
Right-left discrimination	**UNEXPECTED:** Unable to identify right and left sides of own body (5 years).
Two-point discrimination	**UNEXPECTED:** Difficulty in localizing and discriminating when touched in one or two places (6 years).
Graphesthesia	**UNEXPECTED:** Unable to identify geometric shapes drawn in child's open hand (8 years).
Stereognosis	**UNEXPECTED:** Unable to identify common objects placed in own hand (5 years).

Modified from Smith and McNamara, 1984.

SAMPLE DOCUMENTATION

Subjective. A 48-year-old man presents for his annual physical examination. No complaints of poor balance, loss of sensation, unsteady gait. History of diabetes mellitus type 1 for 30 years, well controlled.

Objective. Cranial nerves I to XII grossly intact. Gait is coordinated and even. Romberg test negative. Rapid alternating movements coordinated and smooth. Superficial touch, pain, vibratory sensation are intact bilaterally. Deep tendon reflexes 2+ bilaterally in all extremities. Babinski (plantar) reflex produces expected plantar flexion of toes. No ankle clonus. Monofilament test reveals decreased sensation on plantar surfaces of both feet.

HEAD-TO-TOE EXAMINATION: ADULT

COMPONENTS OF THE EXAMINATION

Because there is no one correct way to order the parts of the physical examination, you are encouraged to consider and then to adapt and edit the following suggested approach for a particular setting, patient condition, or patient disability.

GENERAL INSPECTION

Start examination the moment the patient is within your view. As you first observe patient, for example, in the waiting room, take note of following:

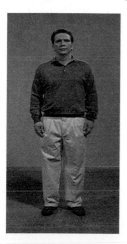

Signs of distress or disease
Habitus
Manner of sitting
Degree of relaxation on face
Relationship with others in room
Degree of interest in what is happening in room

On greeting patient, assess following:
Alacrity with which you are met
Moistness of palm when you shake hands
Eyes—luster and expression of emotion
Skin color
Facial expression
Mobility:
    Use of assistive devices
    Gait
    Sitting, rising from chair
    Taking off coat
Dress and posture
Speech pattern, disorders, foreign language
Difficulty hearing, assistive devices
Stature and build
Musculoskeletal deformities
Vision problems, assistive devices
Eye contact with you
Orientation, mental alertness
Nutritional state
Respiratory problems
Significant others accompanying patient

PATIENT INSTRUCTIONS

Empty bladder.
Remove as much clothing as is necessary (always respecting modesty).
Put on a gown.

MEASUREMENTS

Measure height.
Measure weight.
Assess distance vision—Snellen chart.
Document vital signs—temperature, pulse, respiration, blood pressure
    in both arms.

PATIENT SEATED, WEARING GOWN

Stand in front of patient seated on examining table.

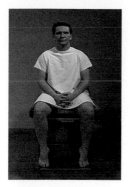

Head and face

Inspect skin characteristics.

Inspect symmetry and external characteristics of eyes and ears.

Inspect configuration of skull.

Inspect and palpate scalp and hair for texture, distribution, quantity of hair.

Palpate facial bones.

Palpate temporomandibular joint while patient opens and closes mouth.

Palpate sinus regions; if tender, transilluminate.

Inspect ability to clench teeth, squeeze eyes tightly shut, wrinkle forehead, smile, stick out tongue, puff out cheeks (cranial nerve [CN] V, CN VII).

Test light sensation of forehead, cheeks, chin (CN V).

Eyes

External examination:

Inspect eyelids, eyelashes, palpebral folds.

Determine alignment of eyebrows.

Inspect sclerae, conjunctivae, irides.

Palpate lacrimal apparatus.

Near-vision screening—Rosenbaum chart (CN II).

Eye function:

Test pupillary response to light and accommodation.

Perform cover-uncover test and light reflex.

Test extraocular eye movements (CN III, CN IV, CN VI).

Assess visual fields (CN II).

Test corneal reflexes (CN V).

Ophthalmoscopic examination:

Test red reflex.

Inspect lens.

Inspect disc, cup margins, vessels, retinal surface, vitreous humor.

Ears

Inspect alignment and placement.

Inspect surface characteristics.

Palpate auricle.

Assess hearing with whisper test (CN VIII).

Perform otoscopic examination:

Inspect canals.

Inspect tympanic membranes for landmarks, deformities, inflammation.

Use a tuning fork to assess bone and air conduction.

Nose

Note structure, position of septum.

Determine patency of each nostril.

Inspect mucosa, septum, turbinates with nasal speculum.

Assess olfactory function when indicated: test sense of smell (CN I).

Mouth and pharynx

Inspect lips, buccal mucosa, gums, hard and soft palates, floor of mouth for color and surface characteristics.

Inspect oropharynx: note anteroposterior pillars, uvula, tonsils, posterior pharynx, mouth odor.

Inspect teeth for color, number, surface characteristics.

Inspect tongue for color, characteristics, symmetry, movement (CN XII).

Test gag reflex and "ah" reflex (CN IX, CN X).

Perform sense of taste test (CN VII, CN IX) when indicated.

Neck

Inspect for symmetry and smoothness of neck and thyroid.

Inspect for jugular venous distention.

Perform active and passive range of motion; test resistance against examiner's hand.

Test strength of shoulder shrug (CN XI).

Palpate carotid pulses. Be sure to palpate one side at a time.

Palpate tracheal position.

Palpate thyroid.

Palpate lymph nodes—preauricular and postauricular, occipital, tonsillar, submental, submandibular, superficial cervical chain, posterior cervical, deep cervical, supraclavicular.

Auscultate carotid arteries and thyroid.

Upper extremities

Observe and palpate hands, arms, shoulders.

Skin and nail characteristics

Muscle mass
Muscular strength
Musculoskeletal deformities
Joint range of motion—fingers, wrists, elbows, shoulders
Assess pulses—radial, brachial.
Palpate epitrochlear nodes.

PATIENT SEATED, BACK EXPOSED

Stand behind patient seated on examining table.
Have males pull gown down to the waist so entire chest and back are exposed.
Have females expose back; keep breasts covered.

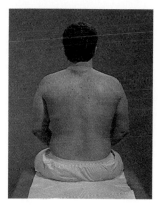

Back and posterior chest

Inspect skin and thoracic configuration.
Inspect symmetry of shoulders, musculoskeletal development.
Inspect and palpate scapulae and spine.
Palpate and percuss costovertebral angle.

Lungs

Inspect respiration—excursion, depth, rhythm, pattern.
Palpate for expansion and tactile fremitus.
Palpate scapular and subscapular nodes.
Percuss posterior chest and lateral walls systematically for resonance.
Percuss for diaphragmatic excursion.
Auscultate systematically for breath sounds (egophony, bronchophony, whispered pectoriloquy): note characteristics and adventitious sounds.

PATIENT SEATED, CHEST EXPOSED

Move around to front of patient.
Have females lower gown to expose anterior chest.

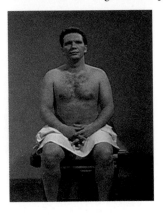

Anterior chest, lungs, heart

Inspect skin, musculoskeletal development, symmetry.
Inspect respirations—patient posture, respiratory effort.
Inspect for pulsations or heaving.
Palpate chest wall for stability, crepitation, tenderness.
Palpate precordium for thrills, heaves, pulsations.
Palpate left chest to locate apical impulse.
Palpate for tactile fremitus.
Palpate nodes—infraclavicular, axillary.
Percuss systematically for breath sounds.
Auscultate systematically for breath sounds.
Auscultate systematically for heart sounds—aortic area, pulmonic area,
    second pulmonic area, tricuspid area, mitral area.

Female breasts

Inspect in these positions—patient's arms extended over head, pushing
    hands on hips, hands pushed together in front of chest, patient
    leaning forward.
Palpate (firmly but gently) breasts in all four quadrants, tail of Spence,
    over areolae; if breasts are large, perform bimanual palpation.
Palpate nipple: compress to observe for discharge.

Male breasts

Inspect breasts and nipples for symmetry, enlargement, surface
    characteristics.
Palpate breast tissue.

PATIENT RECLINING 45 DEGREES

Assist patient to a reclining position at a 45-degree angle.
Stand to side of patient that allows greatest comfort.
Inspect chest in recumbent position.
Inspect jugular venous pulsations; measure jugular venous pressure.

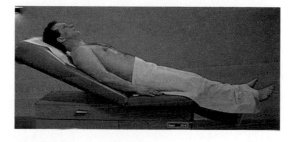

PATIENT SUPINE, CHEST EXPOSED

Assist patient into supine position.
If patient cannot tolerate lying flat, maintain head elevation at 30-degree angle.
Uncover chest while keeping abdomen and lower extremities draped.

Female breasts

Inspect and palpate with patient in recumbent position.
Palpate systematically with patient's arm over her head and with her arm at her side.

Heart

Palpate chest wall for thrills, heaves, pulsations.
Auscultate systematically; turn patient slightly to left side and repeat auscultation.

PATIENT SUPINE, ABDOMEN EXPOSED

Have patient remain supine.
Cover chest with patient's gown.
Arrange draping to expose abdomen from pubis to epigastrium.

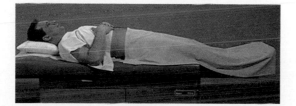

Abdomen

Inspect skin characteristics, contour, pulsations, movement.

Auscultate all quadrants for bowel sounds.

Auscultate aorta and renal, iliac, and femoral arteries for bruits or venous hums.

Percuss all quadrants for tone.

Percuss liver borders and estimate span.

Percuss left midaxillary line for splenic dullness.

Lightly palpate all quadrants at first, then with moderate pressure.

Deeply palpate all quadrants.

Palpate right costal margin for liver border.

Palpate left costal margin for spleen.

Palpate for right and left kidneys.

Palpate midline for aortic pulsation.

Test abdominal reflexes.

Have patient raise head as you inspect abdominal muscles.

Inguinal area

Palpate for lymph nodes, pulses, hernias.

External genitalia, males

Inspect penis, urethral meatus, scrotum, pubic hair.

Palpate scrotal contents (you may want to have patient assume an alternate position, such as standing or sitting).

PATIENT SUPINE, LEGS EXPOSED

Have patient remain supine.

Arrange drapes to cover abdomen and pubis and to expose lower extremities.

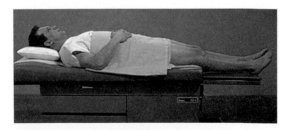

Feet and legs

Inspect for skin characteristics, hair distribution, muscle mass, musculoskeletal configuration.

Palpate for temperature, texture, edema, pulses (dorsalis pedis, posterior tibial, popliteal).

Test range of motion and strength of toes, feet, ankles, knees.

Hips

Palpate hips for stability.
Test range of motion and strength of hips.

PATIENT SITTING, LAP DRAPED

Assist patient to a sitting position.
Have patient wear gown with a drape across lap.

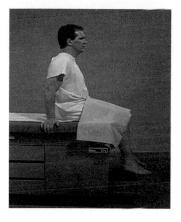

Musculoskeletal

Observe patient moving from lying to sitting position.
Note coordination, use of muscles, muscle strength, ease of movement.

Neurologic

Test sensory function—dull and sharp sensation of forehead, cheeks, chin, lower arms, hands, lower legs, feet.
Test vibratory sensation of wrists, ankles.
Test two-point discrimination of palms, thighs, back.
Test stereognosis, graphesthesia.
Test fine motor function, coordination, and position sense of upper extremities, asking patient to do following:
  Touch nose with alternating index fingers.
  Rapidly alternate touching fingers to thumb.
  Rapidly move index finger between own nose and examiner's finger.
Test fine motor function, coordination, and position sense of lower extremities, asking patient to do following:
  Run heel down tibia of opposite leg.
  Alternately and rapidly cross leg over opposite knee.

Test deep tendon reflexes and compare bilaterally—biceps, triceps, brachioradial, patellar, Achilles.
Test plantar reflex bilaterally.

PATIENT STANDING

Assist patient to standing position.
Stand next to patient.

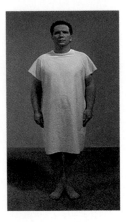

Spine

Inspect and palpate spine as patient bends over at waist.
Test range of motion—hyperextension, lateral bending, rotation of upper trunk.

Neurologic

Observe gait.
Test proprioception and cerebellar function:
    Perform Romberg test.
    Ask patient to walk heel to toe.
    Ask patient to stand on one foot, then the other, with eyes closed.
    Ask patient to hop in place on one foot, then other.
    Ask patient to do deep knee bends.

Abdominal/genital

Test for inguinal and femoral hernias.

FEMALE PATIENT, LITHOTOMY POSITION

Assist female patient into lithotomy position, and drape appropriately.
Sit at end of examining table.

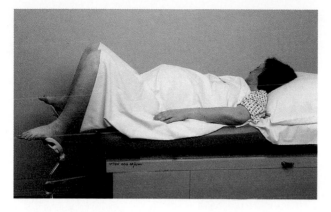

External genitalia

Inspect pubic hair, labia, clitoris, urethral opening, vaginal opening, perineal and perianal area, anus.

Palpate labia and Bartholin glands; milk Skene glands.

Internal genitalia

Perform speculum examination:
    Inspect vagina and cervix.
    Collect Pap smear and other necessary specimens.
Perform bimanual palpation to assess for characteristics of vagina, cervix, uterus, adnexa.
Perform rectovaginal examination to assess rectovaginal septum, broad ligaments.
Perform rectal examination:
    Assess anal sphincter tone and surface characteristics.
    Obtain rectal culture if needed.
    Note characteristics of stool when gloved finger is removed.

MALE PATIENT, BENDING FORWARD

Assist male patient in leaning over examining table or into knee-chest position. Stand behind patient.
Inspect sacrococcygeal and perianal areas.
Perform rectal examination:
    Palpate sphincter tone and surface characteristics.
    Obtain rectal culture if needed.
    Palpate prostate gland and seminal vesicles.
    Note characteristics of stool when gloved finger is removed.

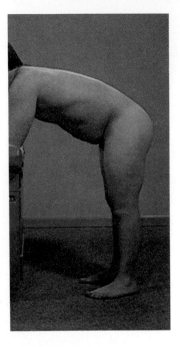

EXAMINATION CONCLUSION

Allow patient to dress in private.

Share findings and interpretations with patient.

Answer any of patient's additional questions.

Confirm that patient has a clear understanding of all aspects of the situation.

If patient is examined in a hospital bed:

Put everything back in order when finished.

Make sure patient is comfortably settled in an appropriate manner.

Put bed side rails up if clinical condition warrants it.

Make sure buttons and buzzers are within easy reach.

SPECIAL CONSIDERATIONS FOR THE HANDICAPPED PATIENT

Each disability affects each patient differently. The familiar process of physical examination must be adapted to constraints imposed by the patient's handicap.

The patient has learned the best way to be transferred from a wheelchair or bed to another site or to a different position. Consult patient about it.

Let the patient who is hearing-, speech-, or vision-impaired guide you to the best communication system for your mutual purposes.

Bowel and bladder concerns are common to many disabled people and should be given the necessary attention during the examination process.

The Healthy Female Evaluation

Following are items to consider for inclusion as part of a routine well-woman visit. This is not intended as an all-inclusive list. Some items may vary depending on the woman's age, health status, and particular risk factors. Past medical history (PMH) and review of systems (ROS) may also be appropriate if indicated. Age and risk-status guidelines for preventive services are available from a variety of sources and authorities.[*]

HISTORY

HISTORY OF PRESENT ILLNESS (HPI)

Age
Last normal menstrual period (LNMP)
Menopause—age achieved, symptoms
Obstetric history—number of pregnancies, term pregnancies, preterm pregnancies, abortions/miscarriages, living children (GPTAL)
Contraceptive measures and history
Sexual history
Breast lumps, discharge, pain, skin changes
Unusual vaginal bleeding or discharge
Abdominal or pelvic pain
Urinary symptoms

---

[*]U.S. Preventive Services Task Force: *Guide to clinical preventive services,* ed 2, Washington, DC, 1996, The Task Force; U.S. Department of Health and Human Services: *Clinician's handbook of preventive services,* Washington, DC, 1994, The Department.
New Releases in Preventive Services. U.S. Preventive Services Task Force. Agency for Healthcare Research and Quality, Rockville, MD. March 2005. http://www.ahrq.gov/clinic/prevnew.htm.
Authorities that produce prevention guidelines include Academy of Family Physicians, American Cancer Society, American College of Obstetricians and Gynecologists, American College of Physicians, American Geriatrics Society, Canadian Task Force on the Periodic Health Examination, National Cancer Institute, and U.S. Preventive Services Task Force.

RISK ASSESSMENT

Cardiovascular—smoking, hypertension, diet, body mass index (BMI), exercise, family history

Cancer—personal/family history of breast, ovarian, or colon cancer; history of sun exposure

Infection—sexually transmitted infection (STI) exposure; tuberculosis exposure; hepatitis vaccine or exposure; last tetanus immunization

Metabolic—calcium supplement, family history of osteoporosis; exercise; personal/family history of diabetes mellitus; hearing impairment in older adults

Injury—alcohol, seat belts, guns, family violence

Mental health—depression: vegetative symptoms (eating, sleeping, concentration, energy, social interaction)

HEALTH HABITS

Breast self-awareness or self-examination

Pap smear—how often, date of last Pap smear; results, ever an abnormal result

Mammogram—date, result of last mammogram

Diet—fat, cholesterol, calcium

Exercise

Smoking

Alcohol/drugs

PHYSICAL EXAMINATION

Vital signs

Height and weight; BMI

Skin—lesions, moles

Lungs

Cardiovascular and peripheral vascular

Breasts—contour, masses, nipple discharge, skin changes

Lymph—regional lymphadenopathy (infraclavicular and supraclavicular, axillary, inguinal)

Abdomen—bowel sounds, masses, organ enlargement, hernias

Pelvic—lesions, discharge; Bartholin glands, urethra, Skene glands; vagina, cervix, adnexa, uterus; rectovaginal septum

Rectal—hemorrhoids, masses, lesions

SCREENING RECOMMENDATIONS

Cardiovascular
    Blood pressure—begin at age 18
    Lipid profile—begin at age 45
Cancer
    Pap smear—begin if sexually active or no later than age 21; frequency
        depends on age, sexual status, PMH, Pap smear history
    Mammogram—begin at age 40; earlier if at increased risk; frequency
        depends on personal and family history, past results
    Fecal occult blood test or flexible sigmoidoscopy or colonoscopy—
        begin at age 50; earlier depending on personal and family history
Infection
    STI testing—depending on exposure status
    TB skin testing—depending on risk status
Metabolic
    BMI for obesity
    Bone density—women aged 65 or older; begin at age 60 if at increased
        risk
    Hearing impairment—older adults
Injury
    Family violence
Mental health
    Alcohol and substance abuse screening
    Depression screening

AGE-SPECIFIC EXAMINATION: INFANTS, CHILDREN, AND ADOLESCENTS

EXAMINATION GUIDELINES

A pediatric physical examination must, of course, be age appropriate. Not every observation must be made on every child at every examination. What you do depends on the individual circumstance and your clinical judgment, each step dependent on the patient's age, physical condition, and emotional state. The order of the examination can be modified according to need. There is no one right way. The safety of the child on the examining table must be ensured. During most of infancy and into the pre–elementary school years (and even later), an adult's lap is most often a better site for much and often all of the examination.

Your notes should include a description of child's behavior during interactions with parent (or surrogate) and with you.

Offer toys or paper and pencil to entertain child (if age appropriate), to develop rapport, and to evaluate development, motor and neurologic status. Attempt to gain child's cooperation, even if it takes more time; future visits will be more pleasant for both of you.

Only if absolutely necessary, restrain child for funduscopic, otoscopic, oral examinations; restraint is easier on an adult lap with the aid of the adult.

Lessen fear of these examinations by permitting child to handle instruments, blow out light, or use them on a doll, a parent, or you.

Take and record temperature, weight, length or height; also, blood pressure (record extremity or extremities used, size of cuff, and method used).

Note percentiles for all measurements.

If clinical issues require it, include arm span, upper segment measurement (crown to top of symphysis), lower segment measurement (symphysis to soles of feet), upper/lower segment ratio, head and chest circumference.

Use a developmental screening test such as Denver II to evaluate language, motor coordination, social skills.

Evaluate mental status as child interacts with you and parent.

CHILD PLAYING

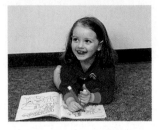

While child plays on the floor, evaluate musculoskeletal and neurologic system while developing a rapport with child.

Observe child's spontaneous activities.

Ask child to demonstrate skills such as throwing a ball, building block towers, drawing geometric figures, coloring.

Evaluate gait, jumping, hopping, range of motion.

Muscle strength: Observe child climbing on parent's lap, stooping, and recovering.

CHILD ON PARENT'S LAP

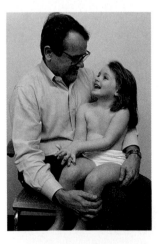

Perform examination on parent's lap; the adult and the patient generally enjoy the experience more and you will find it easier than the examining table.

Begin with child sitting and undressed except for diaper or underpants.

Upper extremities

Inspect arms for movement, size, shape; observe use of hands; inspect hands for number and configuration of fingers, palmar creases.
Palpate radial pulses.
Elicit biceps and triceps reflexes.
Take blood pressure at this point or later.

Lower extremities

Child may stand for much or part of examination.
Inspect legs for movement, size, shape, alignment, lesions.
Inspect feet for alignment, longitudinal arch, number of toes.
Palpate femoral and dorsalis pedis pulses.
Elicit plantar, Achilles, and patellar reflexes.

Head and neck

Inspect head.
Inspect shape, alignment with neck, hairline, position of auricles.
Palpate anterior fontanel for size; head for sutures, depressions; hair for texture.
Measure head circumference.
Inspect neck for webbing, voluntary movement.
Palpate neck: thyroid, muscle tone, lymph nodes, position of trachea.

Chest, heart, lungs

Inspect chest for symmetry, respiratory movement, size, shape, precordial movement, deformity, nipple and breast development.
Palpate anterior chest, locate point of maximal impulse, note tactile fremitus in talking or crying child.
Auscultate anterior, lateral, and posterior chest for breath sounds; count respirations.
Auscultate all cardiac listening areas for S_1 and S_2, splitting, murmurs; count apical pulse.

CHILD RELATIVELY SUPINE, STILL ON LAP, DIAPER LOOSENED

Inspect abdomen.
Auscultate for bowel sounds.
Palpate: identify size of liver and any other palpable organs or masses.
Percuss.
Palpate femoral pulses; compare with radial pulses.
Palpate for inguinal lymph nodes.
Inspect external genitalia.
Males: Palpate scrotum for descent of testes and other masses; crossing the legs in the tailor position helps bring testes down.

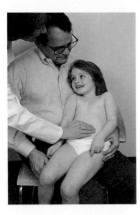

CHILD STANDING

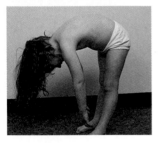

Inspect spinal alignment as child bends slowly forward to touch toes.
Observe posture from anterior, posterior, lateral views.
Observe gait.

CHILD ON PARENT'S LAP

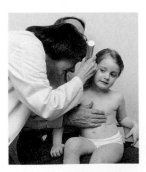

The following steps, often delayed to the end of the examination by many, are particularly more easily performed with a child of appropriate age sitting on a parent's or surrogate's lap:

Inspect eyes: Corneal light reflex, red reflex, extraocular movements, funduscopic examination.

Perform otoscopic examination. Note position and description of pinnae.

Inspect nasal mucosa.

Inspect mouth and pharynx. Note number of teeth, deciduous or permanent, and any special characteristics.

NOTE: By the time child is of school age, it is usually possible to use an examination sequence very similar to that for adults.) See pp. 290-300 for examples of forms used to chart physical growth.

AGE-SPECIFIC ANTICIPATED OBSERVATIONS AND GUIDELINES[*]

Keep in mind that this is a suggested outline, always modified by human variation, and that all percentages are subject to gaussian distribution. History taking can be facilitated by referring to baby books, report cards, pictures, and other materials the family may have at home. Also, these suggestions assume a continuing relationship with the patient. Of course, you must optimally begin with a full history and physical examination when you first see the patient (at whatever age).

2 WEEKS OF AGE

History (particular attention)

Pertinent perinatal history
Social: Sleeping arrangements, housing
Stool pattern
Umbilicus: Healing, discharge, granulation
Diet: Feeding modality, schedule

Development: By this age

80% will lift and turn head when in prone position
40% will follow an object to midline visually

---

*Adapted from clinic forms used in the Primary Care Continuity Clinic in the Children's Medical Center at The Johns Hopkins Hospital under the leadership of Drs. Janet Servint and Kevin Johnson and from the pediatric section, authored by Henry M. Seidel, of "Clinical History and Physical Examination," a booklet prepared for second-year medical students at The Johns Hopkins School of Medicine under the direction of Lawrence S. C. Griffith, MD.

35% will vocalize, become quiet in response to a voice
45% will regard a face intently, diminishing activity for the moment

Physical examination (particular attention)

Establish growth curves (weight, height, head circumference).
Examine hips.
Test reflexes: Moro, root, grasp, step.

Anticipatory guidance (particular attention)

Sleep (emphasize supine position and avoidance of soft and fuzzy threats
to safe breathing)
Feeding: Use of pacifier (need to suck)
Use of bulb syringe (nasal stuffiness)
Safety: Falling, crib sides, car seats
Skin care
Clothing
Illness: Temperature taking
Crying (holding the baby)

Plans and problems

What risks have revealed themselves as you got to know the family?
What are apparent problems? Start a problem list and make appro-
priate dispositions.
Consider need for hemoglobin or hematocrit value.
Consider immunization needs and, throughout, attempt to follow
American Academy of Pediatrics guidelines; on each visit, discuss
benefits, risks, side effects of immunizations (always remember risks
for the immunocompromised).

2 MONTHS OF AGE

History (particular attention)

Expressions of parental concern
Child's apparent temperament
Sleep cycle
Feeding patterns, frequency
Stooling pattern, frequency, color, consistency, straining
Be certain there is no probability of immunocompromise in patient or rele-
vant family members or other contacts (before starting immunizations)
Social issues:
Father's involvement
Living conditions
Smoking, other concerning habits
Any apparent high-risk concerns

Development: By this age

Gross motor:
    80% will lift head to 45 degrees in prone position
    45% will lift head to as much as 90 degrees in prone position
    25% will roll over stomach to back
Fine motor:
    99%+ will follow a moving object to midline
    85% will follow a moving object past midline
Language:
    Almost all will diminish activity at the sound of a voice
    35% will spontaneously vocalize
    Many will vocalize responsively
Psychosocial:
    Almost all will diminish activity when regarding a face
    Almost all will respond to a friendly, cooing face with a social smile
    50% may smile spontaneously or even laugh aloud

Physical examination (particular attention)

Growth curves (weight, height, head circumference)
Hearing
Vision
Hips

Anticipatory guidance

Feeding (delay or at least downplay solids; avoid citrus, wheat, mixed foods, eggs; minimize water)
When and if mother returns to work
Hiccups
Straining at stool
Visual and auditory stimulus (mobiles, mirrors, rattles, singing and talking to baby)
Sibling rivalry (if there are siblings)
Babysitters (checking references, ensuring immunization status, reliability)
Safety (rolling over, playpen, car seat, discourage walker, no smoking)
Sleep (reemphasize location and supine position)
Smoking and contribution to poor health

Plans and problems

Review immunizations and implement as appropriate.
List problems (e.g., allergies, medications, any areas of concern), and make appropriate plans and, if necessary, referrals.
Consider need for hemoglobin or hematocrit value.

4 MONTHS OF AGE

History (particular attention)

Parental concerns
Infant's sleep cycle and temperament
Feeding patterns, frequency, mother's feelings if she is breast-feeding
Stooling pattern, frequency, color, consistency, straining
Social issues:
    Father's involvement
    Amplification of early impressions of home's social structure
    Smoking, other concerning habits
    Any apparent high-risk concerns

Development: By this age

Gross motor:
    80%, when prone, will lift chest up with arm support
    80% will roll over from stomach to back
    35% will have no head lag when pulled to sitting position, and many
        will then hold head steady when kept in that position
Fine motor:
    60% will reach for a dangling object
    Almost all will bring hands together
    Almost all will follow a face or object up to 180 degrees
Language:
    Almost all will laugh aloud
    20% will appear to initiate vocalization
Psychosocial:
    80% will smile spontaneously
    Many will regard their own hand for several seconds

Physical examination (particular attention)

Update growth curves (weight, height, head circumference).
Reassess hearing.
Reassess vision.

Anticipatory guidance

Introduction of solid food (cereal)
Stool changes with changes in diet
Drooling and teething
Thumb sucking, pacifiers, bottles at bedtime
Safety (aspiration, rolling over, holding baby with hot liquids,
    reemphasize earlier discussions [e.g., car seat])
Reemphasis on environmental stimulus
Further discussion of babysitters
Use of antipyretics (e.g., acetaminophen)

Plans and problems

Review immunizations and implement as appropriate.

Maintain problem list, making appropriate plans and, if necessary, referrals.

Consider need for hematocrit or hemoglobin value.

6 MONTHS OF AGE

History (interim details)

Parental concerns

Sleep patterns

Diet

Stooling pattern

Further exploration of social issues

If either parent has not attended these care visits regularly, encourage his or her participation, and address relevant issues

Development: By this age

Gross motor:

    90%, pulled to a sitting position, will have no head lag

    60% will sit alone

    75% will bear some weight on legs

    Almost all will roll over

Fine motor:

    More than half will pass a toy from hand to hand

    60%, in a sitting position, will look for a toy

    40%, in a sitting position, will take two cubes

Language:

    60% will turn toward a voice

    30% will initiate speech sounds (e.g., *mama, dada*) but not specifically

Psychosocial:

    30% may cry and turn away from strangers

    40% may put an object in mouth to explore it, may feed self

    60% may resist an attempt to pull away an object while holding it

Physical examination (particular attention)

Update growth curves.

Double-check hearing and vision.

Look for any new findings, and recheck the old.

Anticipatory guidance

Bedtime routines (discuss putting child to bed while child is awake; waking up at night)

Fear of strangers

Separation anxiety

Safety (begin discussions about what toddlers can get into, cabinets, hot water, electrical outlets, medications and other poisons; inform about local poison control center, syrup of ipecac)

Shoes, when and if to use them

Teething, oral hygiene

Offering a cup

Checking fluoride intake

Addition of solid foods

Plans and problems

Review immunizations and implement as appropriate.

Consider need for a serum lead level, hemoglobin or hematocrit value.

Maintain problem list, making appropriate plans and, if necessary, referrals.

9 MONTHS OF AGE

History (interim details)

Parental concerns

Continued attention to sleep, diet, stooling patterns

Continuing attention to social issues

Development: By this age

Gross motor:
    Almost 100% will sit alone
    80% will stand alone
    45% will cruise
    Some will have begun competent crawling
Fine motor:
    70% will have thumb-finger grasp
    60% will bang two cubes together
    Almost all will finger feed
Language:
    75% will imitate speech sounds
    75% will use *mama, dada* nonspecifically
Psychosocial:
    Almost 100% will try to get to a toy that is out of reach
    85% will play repetitive games (e.g., peek-a-boo)
    45% will be shy with strangers and may cry

Physical examination (particular attention)

Update growth curves.

Constantly reassess earlier findings, and look for anything new.

Anticipatory guidance

Oral hygiene—for example, water without sugar in bottles (avoid tooth decay)

Sleep and desirability of routine (naps, separation anxiety and how to deal with it)

Reemphasis on babysitters, references and reliability

Safety—for example, stair gates and toddlers, falls, poisoning, burns, aspiration (never enough emphasis on safety, smoking, etc.)

Weaning, breast and/or bottle

Uses of discipline

Plans and problems

Review immunizations and implement as appropriate.

Consider need for a serum lead level, hemoglobin or hematocrit value.

Maintain problem list, making appropriate plans and, if necessary, referrals.

12 MONTHS OF AGE

History (interim details)

Assess parental concerns.

Reassess social and system review.

Development: By this age

Gross motor:
    85% will cruise
    70% will stand alone briefly
    50% will walk to some extent, and more will try it with hands held
Fine motor:
    90% will bang two cubes together
    70% will have a good pincer grasp
Language:
    80% will use *mama* and *dada* specifically
    30% will use as many as three additional words
    Almost all will indulge in immature jargoning
Psychosocial:
    Almost all will respond to parent's presence and voice
    Almost all will wave bye-bye
    85% will play pat-a-cake
    50% will drink from a cup
    About half, perhaps a bit more, will play ball with examiner

Physical examination (particular attention)

Update growth curves.

Continue reassessment.
Evaluate gait if walking has begun.

Anticipatory guidance

Reduced food intake in many (this is expected)
Weaning (especially at night)
Increased use of table food
Dental health, toothbrushing
Toilet training (expectations, attitudes)
Discipline (e.g., limit setting)
Safety (childproofing house, street, lead paint, etc.)

Plans and problems

Review immunizations and implement as appropriate.
Consider need for a serum lead level, hemoglobin or hematocrit value, tuberculosis test.
Maintain problem list, making appropriate plans and, if necessary, referrals.

15 MONTHS OF AGE

History (interim details)

Assess parental concerns.
Reassess social and system review.

Development: By this age

Gross motor:
    Almost all will walk well
    Almost all will stoop to recover an object
    35% will walk up steps with help
Fine motor:
    Almost all will drink from a cup
    Almost all will have a neat pincer grasp
    70% will scribble with crayon
    60% will make a tower with two cubes
Language:
    Almost all will use *mama* and *dada* specifically
    75% will use as many as three additional words
    30% will put two words together
Psychosocial:
    Many more than 50% will play ball with examiner
    50% will try to use a spoon
    45% will try to remove clothing

Physical examination (particular attention)

Update growth curves.

Continued reassessment.

Evaluate gait.

Anticipatory guidance

Negativism and independence

Dental health (visit to a dentist)

Toilet training

Weaning

Discipline (e.g., need for consistency)

Safety (all issues, repetitively)

Plans and problems

Review immunizations and implement as appropriate.

Consider need for a serum lead level, hemoglobin or hematocrit value, tuberculosis test.

Maintain problem list, making appropriate plans and, if necessary, referrals.

18 MONTHS OF AGE

History (interim details)

Assess parental concerns.

Reassess social and system review.

Development: By this age

Gross motor:

　　55% will have begun to walk up stairs without much help

　　70% will have started to walk backward

　　More than that will have tried running with at least some success

　　45% will have tried with some success to kick a ball forward, given the opportunity

Fine motor:

　　80% will scribble if given a crayon

　　80% will make a tower with two cubes

　　About half of those will attempt with some success a tower of as many as four cubes

Language:

　　Almost all will have mature jargoning

　　85% will have at least three words in addition to *mama* and *dada*

　　Many of those will put two words together

　　More than half will respond to a one-step command (e.g., when asked to point to a body part)

Psychosocial:
    Well over half will assist with taking off their clothes
    75% will use a spoon successfully, albeit with some spillage

Physical examination (particular attention)

Update growth curves.
Continue reassessment; search for new findings.
Continue to evaluate gait.

Anticipatory guidance

Sleep (naps, nightmares)
Diet (mealtime battles)
Dental health (toothbrushing, dentist)
Toilet training
Discipline (methods and, again, consistency)
Safety (never enough discussion [e.g., seat belt, street and car, childproofing home])
Self-comforting (masturbation, thumb sucking, favorite blankets and toys)
Child care settings if one is necessary

Plans and problems

Review immunizations and implement as appropriate.
Consider need for serum lead level, hemoglobin or hematocrit value, tuberculosis test.
Maintain problem list, making appropriate plans and, if necessary, referrals.

2 YEARS OF AGE

History (interim details)

Assess parental concerns.
Reassess social and system review.

Development: By this age

Gross motor:
    All should run well
    All should walk up steps of reasonable height without holding on
    90% will kick a ball forward
    80% will throw a ball overhand
    60% will do a little jump
    40% may balance on one foot for 1 to 2 seconds
Fine motor:
    Almost all should scribble with a pencil

90% will make a tower of four cubes

70% will copy a vertical line

Language:

All should point to and name parts of body

85% will readily combine two different words

80% will understand *on* and *under*

75% will name a picture

Psychosocial:

85% will give a toy to mother or other significant person

60% will put on some clothing alone and, often, also remove a garment

50% will play games with others

Physical examination (particular attention)

Update growth curves.

Continue reassessment; search for new findings.

Examine mouth, and count number of teeth.

Anticipatory guidance

Independence (limit setting, temper tantrums)

Peer interaction

Safety (poisons and potential poisons, water temperature, car safety seat use)

Toilet training

Nightmares

Use of a cup for drinking (as much as possible)

Plans and problems

Review immunizations and implement as appropriate.

Consider need for serum lead level, hemoglobin or hematocrit value, dental referral, tuberculosis test.

Maintain problem list, making appropriate plans and, if necessary, referrals.

3 YEARS OF AGE

History (interim details)

Assess parental concerns.

Reassess social and system review.

Development: By this age

Gross motor:

75% will balance on one foot for at least 1 second

75% will negotiate a successful broad jump

40% will balance on one foot for as long as 5 seconds

Fine motor:
    80% will copy a circle in addition to a vertical line
    80% will build a tower of as many as eight cubes
Language:
    Speech is becoming more clearly understood in more than half
    80% will use plurals appropriately
    Almost half will give their first and last names appropriately
Psychosocial:
    90% will put on clothing alone
    75% will play interactive games
    50% will separate from mother or other significant person without
        too much stress
    Many will have begun to wash and dry hands

Physical examination (particular attention)

Update growth curves.
Continue reassessment; search for new findings.
Assess whether teeth are coming in appropriately.

Anticipatory guidance

Degrees of independence (limit setting and encouragement, a fine
    balance), other aspects of discipline
Safety (car seat, guns, strangers)
Personal hygiene (hand washing, toothbrushing, proper use of toilet
    tissue)
Day care

Plans and problems

Review immunizations and implement as appropriate.
Consider need for serum lead level, hemoglobin or hematocrit value,
    tuberculosis test.
Maintain problem list, making appropriate plans and, if necessary,
    referrals.

4 YEARS OF AGE

History (interim details)

Assess parental concerns.
Reassess social and system review.

Development: By this age

Gross motor:
    75% will hop on one foot
    75% will balance on one foot for as long as 5 seconds

65% will be able to imitate a heel-toe walk

Many will have begun to throw overhand

Fine motor:

Almost all will copy a circle and a plus sign

80% will pick longer line of two

50% will begin to draw a person in three parts

Language:

Speech is quite understandable in almost all

95% will give their first and last names

85% will understand *cold, tired, hungry*

80% will identify three of four colors

Psychosocial:

Almost all will play games with other children

70% will dress without supervision

Physical examination (particular attention)

Update growth curves.

Continue reassessment; search for new findings.

Remind that hearing and vision must be evaluated at each visit.

Remind that taking blood pressure is an integral part of physical examination.

Anticipatory guidance

Importance of reading to child frequently

Need for a toddler car seat

Fears and fantasies

Separation (reliance on other adults as time goes by)

Safety (matches and lighters out of reach, strangers, street, window guards)

Personal hygiene (again, importance of frequent toothbrushing)

Plans and problems

Review immunizations and implement as appropriate.

Consider need for serum lead level, hemoglobin or hematocrit value, urinalysis.

Maintain problem list, making appropriate plans, and if necessary, referrals.

5 YEARS OF AGE

History (interim details)

Assess parental concerns.

Reassess social and system review.

Development: By this age

Gross motor:

    Almost all will hop nicely on one foot

    75% will balance on one foot for as long as 10 seconds

    60% will do a heel-toe walk backward reasonably well

Fine motor:

    85% will draw a person in three parts

    65% will draw a person in as many as six parts

    60% will copy a square

Language:

    Almost all will identify four colors

    Almost all will understand *on, under, in front of, behind*

    Well over half will define adequately five of the following eight words—*ball, cake, desk, house, banana, curtain, fence, ceiling*

Psychosocial:

    Almost all will dress without supervision

    Almost all will brush teeth without help

    Almost all will play board and card games

    Almost all will be relaxed when left with a babysitter

    More than half will prepare their own cereal

Physical examination (particular attention)

Update growth curves.

Continue reassessment; search for new findings.

Anticipatory guidance

Reading together

School readiness (plays with others, endures separation from parents)

Chores

Discipline (consistency, praising)

Sex identification, education

Peer interaction

Television

Safety (seat belts, guns, bike helmets, matches, swimming; memorize name, address, phone number)

(It is not usually possible to cover so many topics at one visit, so it is usually necessary to be selective based on your knowledge of the family situation.)

Plans and problems

Review immunizations and implement as appropriate.

Consider need for a tuberculosis test, urinalysis.

Maintain problem list, making appropriate plans and, if necessary, referrals.

ELEMENTARY SCHOOL YEARS (6 TO 12 YEARS OF AGE)

History (interim details)

Parental concerns
Child's concerns
Reassess social and system review
    Attention span
    Behavior at home and in school
    School accomplishments and experience
    Enuresis, encopresis, constipation, nightmares

Development

By this time gross and fine motor problems have most often become apparent (but not always; neurologic examination should not be shortchanged). Language and psychosocial skills can be readily investigated in talks with parents and child and in explorations of school and play experiences. Socialization and developing maturity may have different expressions at home, on the playground, and in school, and when with people of different ages and different degrees of acquaintance. Talks with teachers, report cards, and various drawings and other efforts that the child brings home from school can be very helpful.

Physical examination (particular attention)

Update growth curves.
Continue reassessment; search for new findings.
Begin Tanner stage assessment.

Anticipatory guidance

Parent-child rapport
Need for praise
Responsibility
Safety (seat belts, guns, fire, bike helmets, swimming; memorize name,
    address, phone number)
Allowance
Television
Sex education
Dental care
Adult supervision
Discipline (limit setting)
(*Again, time constraints almost always make it necessary to adjust the menu for anticipatory guidance to your judgment about the family's needs.*)

Plans and problems

Review immunizations and implement as appropriate.

Consider need for a tuberculosis test, urinalysis.

Maintain problem list, making appropriate plans and, if necessary, referrals.

ADOLESCENTS

Remember that we have assumed a continuing relationship with the patient from birth on; real life does not always allow that. If you are seeing a patient for the first time, you must, of course, begin with a full history and physical examination.

History (interim details)

Patient's concerns

Parental concerns

Menstrual history

Use of tobacco, alcohol, street or other drugs

Diet and what guides it

Sexual activity (relationships, masturbation, pregnancy and disease control measures); exact timing for all of this should rely on your assessment of the situation and your judgment; in general, social experience

School experience

Suicidal ideation; always be on the alert, and bring it up when necessary

Update knowledge of home and social structure

Revisit in general social and system review

(An adolescent patient [and some elementary school children] may prefer to be or should be seen alone at times and, as they get older, most often or always. This does not mean, however, that the parents are not involved. Proper balance in this relies on your judgment.)

Development

By this time adolescent's physical, neurologic, and cognitive abilities should be well understood, but nothing should be taken for granted. Conversation with patient, parent or parents, and school officials; school records; and, of course, a careful physical examination should all be helpful.

Physical examination (particular attention)

Update growth curves.

Continue reassessment; search for new findings.

Do Tanner stage assessment.

Assess spinal curvatures, particularly in early adolescent females.

Anticipatory guidance

Puberty and its issues; body image
Sexuality, sexually transmitted disease, contraception
Diet
Tobacco, alcohol, drugs
Risk-taking behavior
Exercise
Safety (guns, seat belts, bike helmets)
Family and other social relationships
Independence and responsibility
School and the future
(Time constraints almost always make it necessary to adjust the menu for anticipatory guidance to your judgment about the adolescent's and/or the family's needs.)

Plans and problems

Review immunizations and implement as appropriate.
Consider need for tuberculosis test, sexually transmitted disease testing, hemoglobin or hematocrit determination, urinalysis, lipid screen.
Maintain problem list, making appropriate plans and, if necessary, referrals.

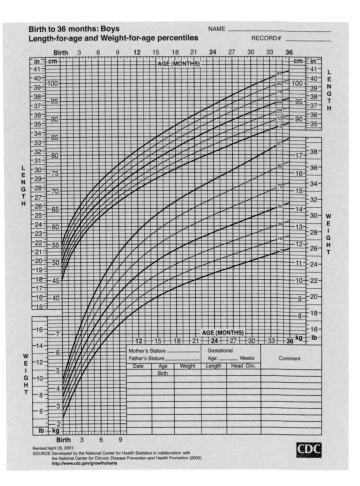

Birth to 36 months: Boys
Length-for-age and Weight-for-age percentiles

NAME _____

RECORD# _____

Revised April 20, 2001.
SOURCE: Developed by the National Center for Health Statistics in collaboration with
the National Center for Chronic Disease Prevention and Health Promotion (2000).
http://www.cdc.gov/growthcharts

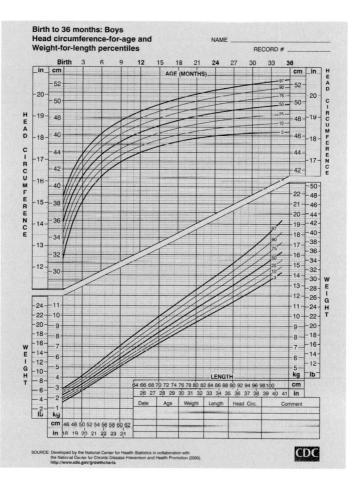

Birth to 36 months: Boys
Head circumference-for-age and
Weight-for-length percentiles

NAME _____

RECORD # _____

SOURCE: Developed by the National Center for Health Statistics in collaboration with
the National Center for Chronic Disease Prevention and Health Promotion (2000).
http://www.cdc.gov/growthcharts

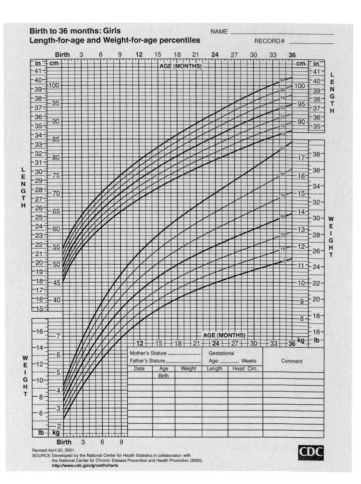

Birth to 36 months: Girls
Length-for-age and Weight-for-age percentiles

NAME

RECORD#

Revised April 20, 2001.
SOURCE: Developed by the National Center for Health Statistics in collaboration with
the National Center for Chronic Disease Prevention and Health Promotion (2000).
http://www.cdc.gov/growthcharts

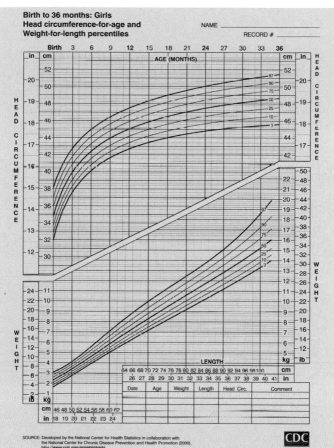

Birth to 36 months: Girls
Head circumference-for-age and
Weight-for-length percentiles

NAME _____

RECORD # _____

SOURCE: Developed by the National Center for Health Statistics in collaboration with
the National Center for Chronic Disease Prevention and Health Promotion (2000).
http://www.cdc.gov/growthcharts

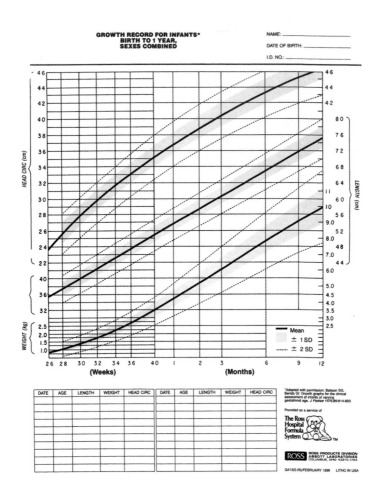

GROWTH RECORD FOR INFANTS*
BIRTH TO 1 YEAR,
SEXES COMBINED

NAME: _____

DATE OF BIRTH: _____

I.D. NO.: _____

DATE	AGE	LENGTH	WEIGHT	HEAD CIRC	DATE	AGE	LENGTH	WEIGHT	HEAD CIRC

*Adapted with permission: Babson SG, Benda GI: Growth graphs for the clinical assessment of infants of varying gestational age. J Pediatr 1976;89:814-820.

Provided as a service of

The Ross Hospital Formula System ™

ROSS ROSS PRODUCTS DIVISION ABBOTT LABORATORIES COLUMBUS, OHIO 43215-1724

G413(0.05)/FEBRUARY 1996   LITHO IN USA

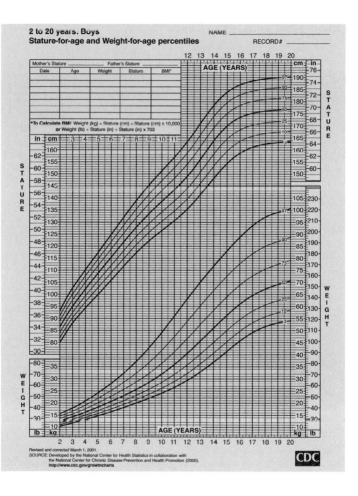

2 to 20 years: Boys
Stature-for-age and Weight-for-age percentiles

NAME _____

RECORD# _____

Revised and corrected March 1, 2001.
SOURCE: Developed by the National Center for Health Statistics in collaboration with
the National Center for Chronic Disease Prevention and Health Promotion (2000).
http://www.cdc.gov/growthcharts

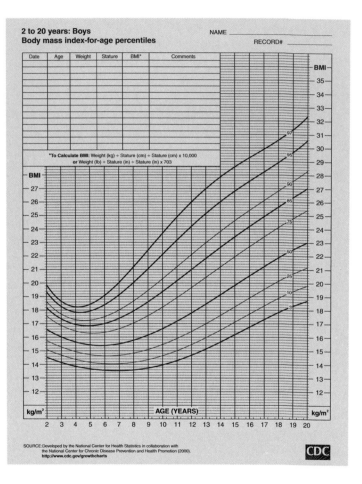

2 to 20 years: Boys
Body mass index-for-age percentiles

NAME
RECORD#

*To Calculate BMI: Weight (kg) ÷ Stature (cm) ÷ Stature (cm) x 10,000
or Weight (lb) ÷ Stature (in) ÷ Stature (in) x 703

SOURCE:Developed by the National Center for Health Statistics in collaboration with
the National Center for Chronic Disease Prevention and Health Promotion (2000).
http://www.cdc.gov/growthcharts

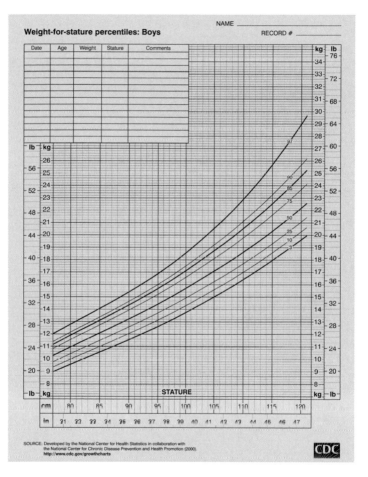

SOURCE: Developed by the National Center for Health Statistics in collaboration with
the National Center for Chronic Disease Prevention and Health Promotion (2000).
http://www.cdc.gov/growthcharts

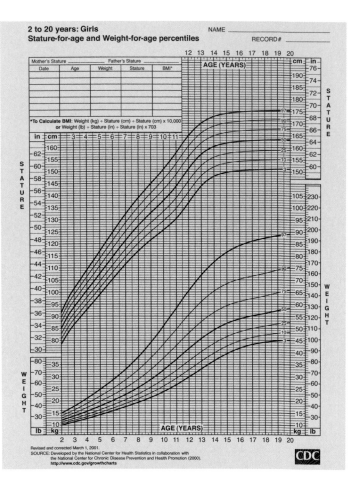

2 to 20 years: Girls
Stature-for-age and Weight-for-age percentiles

NAME _____

RECORD# _____

*To Calculate BMI: Weight (kg) ÷ Stature (cm) ÷ Stature (cm) x 10,000
or Weight (lb) ÷ Stature (in) ÷ Stature (in) x 703

Revised and corrected March 1, 2001.
SOURCE: Developed by the National Center for Health Statistics in collaboration with
the National Center for Chronic Disease Prevention and Health Promotion (2000).
http://www.cdc.gov/growthcharts

CDC

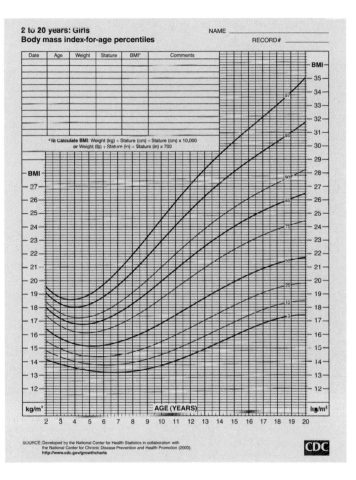

2 to 20 years: Girls
Body mass index-for-age percentiles

NAME _____
RECORD# _____

*To Calculate BMI: Weight (kg) ÷ Stature (cm) ÷ Stature (cm) x 10,000
or Weight (lb) ÷ Stature (in) ÷ Stature (in) x 703

SOURCE: Developed by the National Center for Health Statistics in collaboration with
the National Center for Chronic Disease Prevention and Health Promotion (2000).
http://www.cdc.gov/growthcharts

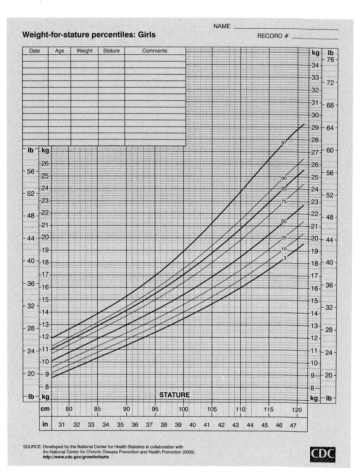

REPORTING AND RECORDING

SUBJECTIVE DATA—THE HISTORY

Subjective data are the positive and negative pieces of information that the patient offers. Record the patient's history, especially during an initial visit, to provide a comprehensive database. Arrange information appropriately in specific categories, usually in a particular sequence such as chronologic order with most recent information first. Include both positive and negative data that contribute to the assessment. Use the following organized sequence as a guide.

IDENTIFYING INFORMATION

Record data recommended by health agency.

Patient's name
Identification number/social security number
Age, sex
Marital status
Address (home and business)
Phone numbers
Occupation, employer
Insurance plan, number
Date of visit
For children and dependent adults, names of parents or next of kin
Put identifying information on each page of record.

SOURCE AND RELIABILITY OF INFORMATION

Document who is providing the history and relationship to patient.
Indicate when an old record is used.
State judgment about reliability of information.

CHIEF COMPLAINT/PRESENTING PROBLEM/REASON FOR SEEKING CARE

Description of patient's main reasons for seeking health care, in patient's own words with quotation marks. Paraphrase only if this makes complaint more clear.

Include duration of problem.

HISTORY OF PRESENT PROBLEM

List and describe current symptoms of chief complaint and their appearance chronologically in reverse order, dating events and symptoms.

List any expected symptoms that are absent.

Identify anyone in household with same symptoms.

Note pertinent information from review of systems, family history, and personal/social history along with findings.

Where more than one problem is identified, address each in a separate paragraph, including the following details of symptom occurrence:

Onset: When problem first started, chronologic order of events, setting and circumstances, manner of onset (sudden versus gradual)

Location: Exact location, localized or generalized, radiation patterns

Duration: How long problem has lasted, intermittent or continuous, duration of each episode

Character: Nature of symptom

Aggravating/associated factors: Food, activity, rest, certain movements; nausea, vomiting, diarrhea, fever, chills, etc.

Relieving factors: Prescribed treatments and/or self-remedies, alternative or complementary therapies, their effect on the problem; food, rest, heat, ice, activity, position, etc.

Temporal factors: Frequency; relation to other symptoms, problems, functions; symptom improvement or worsening over time

Severity of symptoms: Quantify on a 0 to 10 scale; effect on patient's lifestyle

MEDICAL HISTORY

List and describe each of the following with dates of occurrence and any specific information available:

General health and strength over lifetime as patient perceives it; disabilities and functional limitations

Hospitalization and/or surgery: Dates, hospital, diagnosis, complications

Injuries and disabilities

Major childhood illnesses

Adult illnesses and serious injuries

Immunizations: Polio, diphtheria-pertussis-tetanus, tetanus toxoid, *Hemophilus influenza* type b, hepatitis A and B, measles, mumps, rubella, varicella, Prevnar, influenza, anthrax, smallpox, cholera, typhus, typhoid, meningococcal, pneumococcal, bacille Calmette-Guérin (BCG), last purified protein derivative (PPD) or other skin tests, unusual reaction to immunizations

Medications: Past, current, recent medications (prescribed, nonprescription, complementary therapies, home remedies); dosages

Allergies: Drugs, foods, environmental

Transfusions: Reason, date, number of units transfused, reactions

Emotional status: History of mood disorders, psychiatric attention or medications

Recent laboratory tests (e.g., glucose, cholesterol, Pap smear, mammogram, prostate-specific antigen)

Family history

Present information about age and health of family members in narrative or pedigree form, including at least three generations.

Family members: Include parents, grandparents, aunts and uncles, siblings, spouse, children. For deceased family members, note age at time of death and cause, if known.

Major health or genetic disorders: Include hypertension; cancer; cardiac, respiratory, kidney, or thyroid disorders; strokes; asthma or other allergic manifestations; blood dyscrasia; psychiatric difficulties; tuberculosis; diabetes mellitus; hepatitis; or other familial disorders. Note spontaneous abortions and stillbirths.

PERSONAL/SOCIAL HISTORY

Include information according to concerns of patient and influence of health problem on patient's and family's life:

Cultural background and practices, birthplace, position in family

Marital status

Religious preference, religious or cultural proscriptions for medical care

Home conditions: Economic condition, number in household, pets

Occupation: Work conditions and hours, physical or mental strain, protective devices used; exposure to chemicals, toxins, poisons, fumes, smoke, asbestos, or radioactive material at home or work

Environment: Home, school, work; structural barriers if handicapped, community services utilized; travel; exposure to contagious diseases

Current health habits and/or risk factors: Exercise; smoking; salt intake; weight control; diet, vitamins and other supplements; caffeine-containing beverages; alcohol or recreational drug use;

response to CAGE, TACE, or RAFFT questions (see Appendix) related to alcohol use; participation in a drug or alcohol treatment program or support group

Sexual activity: Protection method, contraception

General life satisfaction, hobbies, interests, sources of stress, adolescent's response to HEEADSSS questions (see Appendix)

REVIEW OF SYSTEMS

Organize in general head-to-toe sequence, including an impression of each symptom.

Record expected or negative findings as absence of symptoms or problems.

When unexpected or positive findings are stated by patient, include details from further inquiry as you would in the present illness.

Include the following categories of information (sequence may vary):

General constitutional symptoms
Diet
Skin, hair, nails
Head and neck
Eyes, ears, nose, mouth, throat
Endocrine
Breasts
Heart and blood vessels
Chest and lungs
Hematologic
Lymphatic, immunologic
Gastrointestinal
Genitourinary
Musculoskeletal
Neurologic
Psychiatric

OBJECTIVE DATA—PHYSICAL FINDINGS

Objective data are the findings resulting from direct observation—what you see, hear, and touch.

GENERAL STATEMENT

Age, race, sex, general appearance

Nutritional status, weight, height, frame size, body mass index

Vital signs: Temperature, pulse rate, respiratory rate, blood pressure (two extremities, two positions)

MENTAL STATUS

Physical appearance and behavior
Cognitive: Memory, reasoning, attention span, response to questions
Speech and language: Voice quality, articulation, content, coherence, comprehension
Emotional stability: Anxiety, depression, disturbance in thought content

SKIN

Color, integrity, temperature, hydration, tattoos, scars
Presence of edema, excessive perspiration, unusual odor
Presence and description of lesions (size, shape, location, inflammation, tenderness, induration, discharge), parasites
Hair texture and distribution
Nail configuration, color, texture, condition, presence of clubbing, nail plate adherence, firmness

HEAD

Size and contour of head, scalp appearance and movement
Facial features (characteristics, symmetry)
Presence of edema or puffiness, tenderness
Temporal arteries: Characteristics

EYES

Visual acuity, visual fields
Appearance of orbits, conjunctivae, sclerae, eyelids, eyebrows
Pupillary shape, consensual response to light and accommodation, extraocular movements, corneal light reflex, cover-uncover test
Ophthalmoscopic findings of cornea, lens, retina, optic disc, macula, retinal vessel size, caliber, and arteriovenous crossings

EARS

Configuration, position and alignment of auricles
Otoscopic findings of canals (cerumen, lesions, discharge, foreign body) and tympanic membranes (integrity, color, landmarks, mobility, perforation)
Hearing: Air and bone conduction tests, whispered voice, conversation

NOSE

Appearance of external nose, nasal patency, flaring
Nasal mucosa and septum, color, alignment, discharge, crusting, polyp
Appearance of turbinates

Presence of sinus tenderness or swelling
Discrimination of odors

MOUTH AND THROAT

Number, occlusion and condition of teeth; presence of dental appliances
Lips, tongue, buccal and oral mucosa, floor of mouth (color, moisture, surface characteristics, ulcerations, induration, symmetry)
Oropharynx, tonsils, palate (color, symmetry, exudate)
Symmetry and movement of tongue, soft palate and uvula; gag reflex
Discrimination of taste

NECK

Mobility, suppleness, strength
Position of trachea
Thyroid size, shape, tenderness, nodules
Presence of masses, webbing, skinfolds

CHEST

Size and shape of chest, anteroposterior versus transverse diameter, symmetry of movement with respiration
Presence of retractions, use of accessory muscles, diaphragmatic excursion

LUNGS

Respiratory rate, depth, regularity, quietness or ease of respiration
Palpation findings: Symmetry and quality of tactile fremitus, thoracic expansion
Percussion findings: Quality and symmetry of percussion notes, diaphragmatic excursion
Auscultation findings: Characteristics of breath sounds (pitch, duration, intensity, vesicular, bronchial, bronchovesicular) unexpected breath sounds
Characteristics of cough
Presence of friction rub, egophony, whispered pectoriloquy or bronchophony

BREASTS

Size, contour, venous patterns
Symmetry, texture, masses, scars, tenderness, thickening, nodules, discharge, retraction, or dimpling
Characteristics of nipples and areolae

HEART

Anatomic location of apical impulse
Heart rate, rhythm, amplitude, contour
Palpation findings: Pulsations, thrills, heaves, or lifts
Auscultation findings: Characteristics of S_1 and S_2 (location, intensity, pitch, timing, splitting, systole, diastole)
Presence of murmurs, clicks, snaps, S_3 or S_4 (timing, location, radiation intensity, pitch, quality)

BLOOD VESSELS

Blood pressure: Comparison between extremities with position change
Jugular vein pulsations and distention, pressure measurement
Presence of bruits over carotid, temporal, renal, and femoral arteries, abdominal aorta
Pulses in distal extremities
Temperature, color, hair distribution, skin texture, nail beds of lower extremities
Presence of edema, swelling, vein distention, Homans sign, or tenderness of lower extremities

ABDOMEN

Shape, contour, visible aorta pulsations, venous patterns, hernia
Auscultation findings: Bowel sounds in all quadrants, character
Palpation findings: Aorta, organs, feces, masses, location, size, contour, consistency, tenderness, muscle resistance
Percussion findings: Areas of different percussion notes, costovertebral angle tenderness
Liver span

FEMALE GENITALIA

Appearance of external genitalia and perineum, distribution of pubic hair, inflammation, excoriation, tenderness, scarring, discharge
Internal examination findings: Appearance of vaginal mucosa, cervix, discharge, odor, lesions
Bimanual examination findings: Size, position, tenderness of cervix, vaginal walls, uterus, adnexa, ovaries
Rectovaginal examination findings
Urinary incontinence with bearing down

MALE GENITALIA

Appearance of external genitalia, circumcision status, location and size of urethral opening, smegma, discharge, lesions, distribution of pubic hair

Palpation findings: Penis, testes, epididymides, vasa deferentia, contour, consistency, tenderness

Presence of hernia or scrotal swelling

ANUS AND RECTUM

Sphincter control, presence of hemorrhoids, fissures, skin tags, polyps

Rectal wall contour, tenderness, sphincter tone

Prostate size, contour, consistency, mobility

Color and consistency of stool

LYMPHATIC

Presence of lymph nodes in head, neck, epitrochlear, axillary, or inguinal areas

Size, shape, consistency, warmth, tenderness, mobility, discreteness of nodes

MUSCULOSKELETAL

Posture: Alignment of extremities and spine, symmetry of body parts

Symmetry of muscle mass, tone and muscle strength; grading of strength, fasciculations, spasms

Range of motion, passive and active; presence of pain with movement

Appearance of joints; presence of deformities, tenderness or crepitus

NEUROLOGIC

Cranial nerves: Specific findings for each or specify those tested, if findings are recorded in head and neck sections

Cerebellar and motor function: Gait, balance, coordination with rapid alternating motions

Sensory function, symmetry (touch, pain, vibration, temperature, monofilament)

Superficial and deep tendon reflexes: Symmetry, grade

ASSESSMENT

The assessment section is composed of your interpretations and conclusions, their rationale, the diagnostic possibilities, and present and anticipated problems—what you think.

For each new and existing problem on the problem list make a differential diagnosis list with rationale based on subjective and objective data

Describe disease progression or complication

PLAN

The plan describes the need to invoke diagnostic resources, therapeutic modalities, and other resources and the rationale for these decisions—what you intend to do.

Diagnostic tests ordered or performed

Therapeutic treatment plan

Patient education

Referrals initiated

Future visit to evaluate plan

Appendix

QUICK REFERENCE TO SPECIAL HISTORIES

CAGE Questionnaire: A Framework for Detecting Alcoholism

Mnemonic	Questions
C: Concern, cut down	Have you ever been concerned about your own or someone else's drinking? Have you ever felt the need to cut down on drinking?
	Probe: What was it like? Were you successful? Why did you decide to cut down?
A: Annoyed	Have you ever felt annoyed by criticism of your drinking?
	Probe: What caused the worry or concern? Do you ever get irritated by others' worries? Have you ever limited what you drink to please someone?
G: Guilty	Have you ever felt guilty about your drinking? Have you ever felt guilty about something you said or did while you were drinking?
	Probe: Have you ever been bothered by anything you have done or said while you've been drinking? Have you ever regretted anything that has happened to you while you were drinking?
E: Eye-opener	Have you ever felt the need for a morning eye-opener drink?
	Probe: Have you ever felt shaky or tremulous after a night of heavy drinking? What did you do to relieve the shakiness? Have you ever had trouble getting back to sleep early in the morning after a night of heavy drinking?

From Ewing, 1998.

TACE Questionnaire: A Framework for Prenatal Detection of Risk Drinking

Mnemonic	Questions
T: Take	How many drinks does it take to make you feel high? (More than two drinks suggests a tolerance to alcohol that is a red flag.) How many when you first started drinking? When was that? Which do you prefer: beer, wine, or liquor?
A: Annoyed	Have people annoyed you by criticizing your drinking?
C: Cut down	Have you felt you ought to cut down on your drinking?
E: Eye-opener	Have you ever had an eye-opener drink first thing in the morning to steady your nerves or get rid of a hangover?

A positive answer to T alone or to two of A, C, or E may signal a problem with a high degree of probability, and positive answers to all four, with great certainty.

From Sokol, Martier, Ager, 1989.

The RAFFT Questionnaire: A Framework for Detecting Substance Use Disorders in Adolescents

Mnemonic	Questions
T: Take	How many drinks does it take to make you feel high? (More than two drinks suggests a tolerance to alcohol that is a red flag.) How many when you first started drinking? When was that? Which do you prefer: beer, wine, or liquor?
R: Relax	Do you drink or take drugs to relax, feel better about yourself, or fit in?
A: Alone	Do you ever drink or take drugs while you are alone?
F: Friends	Do any of your closest friends drink or use drugs?
F: Family	Does a close family member have a problem with alcohol or drugs?
T: Trouble	Have you ever gotten into trouble from drinking or taking drugs?

From Bastiaens, Francis, Lewis, 2000.

Domestic Violence: Three Questions as a Brief Screening Instrument

1. Have you been hit, kicked, punched, or otherwise hurt by someone within the past year?
2. Do you feel safe in your current relationship?
3. Is a partner from a previous relationship making you feel unsafe now?

A positive response to any one of the three questions constitutes a positive screen for partner violence.

The first question, which addresses physical violence, has been validated in studies as an accurate measure of 1-year prevalence rates.

The last two questions evaluate the perception of safety and estimate the short-term risk of further violence and the need for counseling, but reliability and validity evaluations have not yet been established.

From Feldhaus et al, 1997.

BATHE Questionnaire: A Framework for Understanding the Patient in the Context of His or Her Total Life Situation

Mnemonic	Questions
B: Background	What is going on in your life?
	What is going on right now?
	Has anything changed recently?
A: Affect	How do you feel about that?
	What is your mood?
T: Trouble	What about the situation troubles you most?
	What worries or concerns you?
H: Handling	How are you handling that?
	How are you coping?
E: Empathy	That must be very difficult for you.
	I can understand that you would feel that way.

From Stuart, Lieberman, 1993; Lieberman, 1997.

HOPE Questionnaire: A Framework for Spiritual Assessment

Mnemonic	Questions
H: Hope— sources of hope, meaning, comfort, strength, peace, love, and connection	We have been discussing your support systems. I was wondering, what is there in your life that gives you internal support?
	What are your sources of hope, strength, comfort, and peace?
	What do you hold on to during difficult times?
	What sustains you and keeps you going?
	For some people, their religious or spiritual beliefs act as a source of comfort and strength in dealing with life's ups and downs; is this true for you?
	If the answer is yes, go on to O and P questions. If the answer is no, consider asking, "Was it ever?" If the answer is yes, ask, "What changed?"

Continued

Mnemonic	Questions
O: Organized religion	Do you consider yourself part of an organized religion? How important is this to you?
	What aspects of your religion are helpful and not so helpful to you?
	Are you part of a religious or spiritual community? Does it help you? How?
P: Personal spirituality/ practices	Do you have personal spiritual beliefs that are independent of organized religion? What are they?
	Do you believe in God? What kind of relationship do you have with God?
	What aspects of your spirituality or spiritual practices do you find most helpful to you personally? (Examples include prayer, meditation, reading scripture, attending religious services, listening to music, hiking, communing with nature.)
E: Effects on medical care and end-of-life issues	Has being sick (or your current situation) affected your ability to do the things that usually help you spiritually (or affected your relationship with God)?
	As a doctor, is there anything that I can do to help you access the resources that usually help you?
	Are you worried about any conflicts between your beliefs and your medical situation/care/decisions?
	Would it be helpful for you to speak to a clinical chaplain/community spiritual leader?
	Are there any specific practices or restrictions I should know about in providing your medical care (e.g., dietary restrictions, use of blood products)?
	If the patient is dying: How do your beliefs affect the kind of medical care you would like me to provide over the next few days/weeks/months?

Anandarajah, Hight, 2001.

SPIRIT Questionnaire: A Framework for Spiritual Assessment

Mnemonic	Questions
S: Spiritual belief system	What is your formal religious affiliation? Name or describe your spiritual belief system.
P: Personal spirituality	Describe the beliefs and practices of your religion or spiritual system that you personally accept.
	Describe the beliefs or practices you do not accept.
	Do you accept or believe (specific tenet or practice)?
	What does your spirituality/religion mean to you?
	What is the importance of your spirituality/religion in daily life?
I: Integration with a spiritual community	Do you belong to any spiritual or religious group or community? What is your position or role?
	What importance does this group have to you? Is it a source of support? In what ways?
	Does or could this group provide help in dealing with health issues?
R: Ritualized practices and restrictions	Are there specific practices that you carry out as part of your religion/spirituality (e.g., prayer or meditation)?
	Are there certain lifestyle activities or practices that your religion/spirituality encourages or forbids? Do you comply?
	What significance do these practices and restrictions have to you?
	Are there specific elements of medical care that you forbid on the basis of religious/spiritual grounds?

Continued

Mnemonic	Questions
I: Implications for medical care	What aspects of your religion/spirituality would you like me to keep in mind as I care for you?
	Would you like to discuss religious or spiritual implications of health care?
	What knowledge or understanding would strengthen our relationship as physician and patient?
	Are there any barriers to our relationship based on religious or spiritual issues?
T: Terminal events planning	As we plan for your care near the end of life, how does your faith affect your decisions?
	Are there particular aspects of care that you wish to forgo or have withheld because of your faith?

From Maugans, 1996.

ETHNIC Questionnaire: A Framework for Culturally Competent Clinical Practice

Mnemonic	Questions
E: Explanation	Why do you think you have these symptoms? What do friends, family, and others say? Do you know others with this problem? Have you seen it on TV, heard about it on the radio, or read about it in the newspaper?
T: Treatment	Do you take any treatments, medicines, or home remedies to treat the illness or to stay healthy? What kinds of treatment are you seeking from me?
H: Healers	Have you sought advice from friends, alternative folk healers, or other nondoctors?
N: Negotiate	Negotiate mutually acceptable options; incorporate patient's beliefs. Ask results patient hopes to achieve from intervention.
I: Intervention	Determine an intervention with your patient. May include incorporation of alternative treatments, spirituality, healers, or other cultural practices (e.g., foods to be eaten or avoided).
C: Collaborate	Collaborate with the patient, family, health team members, healers, and community resources.

Modified from Levin et al, 1997.

The HEEADSSS Psychosocial Interview for Adolescents (Essential Questions)

Mnemonic	Questions
H: Home	Who lives with you? Where do you live? Do you have your own room?
	What are relationships like at home?
	To whom are you closest at home?
	To whom can you talk at home?
	Is there anyone new at home? Has someone left recently?
	Have you moved recently?
	Have you ever had to live away from home? (Why?)
E: Education and employment	What are your favorite subjects at school? Your least favorite subjects?
	How are your grades? Any recent changes? Any dramatic changes in the past?
	Have you changed schools in the past few years?
	What are your future education/ employment plans/goals?
	Are you working? Where? How much?
E: Eating	What do you like and not like about your body?
	Have there been any recent changes in your weight?
	Have you dieted in the last year? How? How often?
	Have you done anything else to try to manage your weight?
	How much exercise do you get in an average day? Week?
	What do you think would be a healthy diet? How does that compare to your current eating patterns?

Mnemonic	Questions
A: Activities	What do you and your *friends* do for fun? (With whom, where, and when?)
	What do you and your *family* do for fun? (With whom, where, and when?)
	Do you participate in any sports or other activities?
	Do you regularly attend a church group, club, or other organized activity?
D: Drugs	Do you and your friends use tobacco? Alcohol? Other drugs?
	Does anyone in your family use tobacco? Alcohol? Other drugs?
	Do you use tobacco? Alcohol? Other drugs?
	Is there any history of alcohol or drug problems in your family? Does anyone at home use tobacco?
S: Sexuality	Have you ever been in a romantic relationship?
	Tell me about the people that you've dated. OR Tell me about your sex life.
	Have any of your relationships ever been sexual relationships?
	Are your sexual activities enjoyable?
	What does the term "safer sex" mean to you?
S: Suicide and depression	Do you feel sad or down more than usual?
	Do you feel yourself crying more than usual?
	Are you "bored" all the time?
	Are you having trouble getting to sleep?
	Have you thought a lot about hurting yourself or someone else?

Continued

Mnemonic	Questions
S: Safety (savagery)	Have you ever been seriously injured? (How?) How about anyone else you know?
	Do you always wear a seatbelt in the car?
	Have you ever ridden with a driver who was drunk or high? When? How often?
	Do you use safety equipment for sports and/or other physical activities (for example, helmets for biking or skateboarding)?
	Is there any violence at your school? In your neighborhood? Among your friends?
	Have you ever been physically or sexually abused? Have you ever been raped, on a date or at any other time? (If not asked previously)

From Goldenring, Rosen, 2004.

References

Adams JA: Evolution of a classification scale: medical evaluation of suspected child sexual abuse, *Child Maltreat* 6:31-36, 2001.

Agency for Healthcare Research and Quality: *Management of acute otitis media: summary, evidence report/technology assessment No. 15,* Rockville, Md, June 2000, The Agency; www.ahrq.gov/clinic/epcsums/otitisum.htm (accessed 11/2005).

Ahuja V, Yencha MW, Lassen LF: Head and neck manifestations of gastroesophageal reflux disease, *Am Fam Physician* 50(3):873-880, 885-886, 1999.

American Academy of Audiology: *Newborn hearing screening,* 2002, www.audiology.org/professional/tech/eihbrochure.php (accessed 11/2005).

American Academy of Pediatrics: Guidelines for the evaluation of sexual abuse of children: subject review (RE 9819), *Pediatrics* 103(1):186-191, 1999.

American Academy of Pediatrics: Committee on Bioethics: informed consent, parental permission, and assent in pediatric practice, *Pediatrics,* 95(2): 314-317, 1995.

American Academy of Pediatrics and American Academy of Family Physicians: *Clinical practice guideline: diagnosis and management of acute otitis media,* 2004, www.aap.org/policy/otitis.htm (accessed 11/2005).

American Academy of Pediatrics Committee on Quality Improvement, Subcommittee on Developmental Dysphasia of the Hip: Clinical practice guideline: early detection of developmental dysphasia of the hip, *Pediatrics* 105(4):896-905, 2000.

American Academy of Pediatrics Committee on Sports Medicine and Fitness: Medical conditions affecting sports participation, *Pediatrics* 107(5): 1205-1209, 2001.

American Cancer Society: *Cancer reference information: prevention and early detection,* www.cancer.org (accessed 11/2005).

Anandarajah G, Hight E: Spirituality and medical practice: using the HOPE questions as a practical tool for spiritual assessment, *Am Fam Physician* 63(1):81-89, 2001.

Apantaku LM: Breast cancer diagnosis and screening, *Am Fam Physician* 62(3):596-602, 2000.

Arvidson CR: The adolescent gynecologic exam, *Pediatr Nurs* 25(1):71-74, 1999.

Athey J, Moody-Williams J: *Serving disaster survivors: achieving cultural competence in crisis counseling,* Washington, DC, 2000, Emergency Services and Disaster Relief Branch, Center for Mental Health Services, Substance Abuse and Mental Health Services Administration.

Attia MW et al: Performance of a predictive model for streptococcal pharyngitis in children, *Arch Pediatr Adolesc Med* 155:687-691, 2001.

Bacal DA, Wilson MC: Strabismus: getting it straight, *Contemp Pediatr* 17:49, 2000.

Baran R, Dawber RPR, Levene G: *Color atlas of the hair, scalp and nails,* St Louis, 1991, Mosby.

Barkauskas VH et al: *Health and physical assessment,* ed 3, St Louis, 2001, Mosby.

Bastiaens L, Francis G, Lewis K: The RAFFT as a screening tool for adolescent substance use disorders, *Am J Addict* 9(1):10-16, 2000.

Bluestone CD, Klein JO: *Otitis media in infants and children,* ed 3, Philadelphia, 2001, WB Saunders.

Boustani M et al: Screening for dementia in primary care: a summary of the evidence for the U.S. Preventive Services Task Force, *Annals Intern Med* 138:927-937, 2003.

Brooke P, Bullock R: Validation of a 6-item cognitive impairment test with a view to primary care, *Int J Geriatr Psychiatry* 14(1):936-940, 1999.

Brown JE, Carlson M: Nutrition and multi-fetal pregnancy, *J Am Diet Assoc* 100(3):343-348, 2000.

Burrow GN: Thyroid diseases. In Burrow GN, Duffy TP, editors: *Medical complications during pregnancy,* ed 5, Philadelphia, 1999, WB Saunders.

Castiglia PT: Depression in children, *J Pediatr Health Care* 14(2):73-75, 2000.

Caulin-Glaser T, Setaro J: Pregnancy and cardiovascular disease. In Burrow GN, Duffy TP, editors: *Medical complications during pregnancy,* ed 5, Philadelphia, 1999, WB Saunders.

Centers for Disease Control and Prevention: *Guideline for isolation precautions in hospitals,* www.cdc.gov/ncidod/hip/isolat/isolat.htm (accessed 4/2005).

Centers for Disease Control and Prevention: *Standard precautions,* www.cdc.gov/ncidod/hip/isolat/std_prec_excerpt.htm (accessed 11/2005).

Centers for Disease Control and Prevention: *Viral hepatitis,* www.cdc.gov/ncidod/diseases/hepatitis/index.htm (accessed 11/2005).

Chelebowski RT et al: Influence of estrogen plus progestin on breast cancer and mammography in healthy postmenopausal women: the Woman's Health Initiative randomized trial, *JAMA* 289:3243-3253, 2003.

Chumlea W et al: Age at menarche and racial comparisons in US girls, *Pediatrics* 111:110-113, 2003; www.pediatrics.org/cgi/content/full/111/1/110 (accessed 11/2005).

D'Arcy CA, McGee S: Does this patient have carpal tunnel syndrome? *JAMA* 283(23):3110-3117, 2000.

Deering CG: To speak or not to speak: self-closure with patients, *Am J Nursing* 99:34-38, 1999.

Delves PJ, Roitt IM: The immune system, *N Engl J Med* 343:108-116, 2000.

Dowd R, Cavalieri RJ: Help your patient live with osteoporosis, *Am J Nursing* 99(4):55-60, 1999.

Edge V, Miller M: *Women's health care,* St Louis, 1994, Mosby.

Ewing JA: Screening for alcoholism using CAGE: cut down, annoyed, guilty, eye opener, *JAMA* 280(2):1904-1905, 1998.

Executive Summary of the Third Report of the National Cholesterol Education Program Expert Panel on Detection, Evaluation, and Treatment of High Blood Cholesterol in Adults (Adult Treatment Panel III), *JAMA* 285(19): 2486-2497, 2001.

Farrar WE et al: *Infectious diseases,* ed 2, London, 1992, Gower.

Feldhaus K et al: Accuracy of 3 brief screening questions for detecting partner violence in the emergency department, *JAMA* 277(17):1357-1361, 1997.

Ferrie B: Complementary modalities in the new millennium, *Advance for Nurses* May 3:28-29, 1999.

Ferro RT, Jain R, McKeag DB, Escobar R: A nonoperative approach to shoulder impingement syndrome. *Advanced Studies in Medicine*, 3(9):518-528, 2003.

Folstein M et al: The meaning of cognitive impairment in the elderly, *J Am Geriatr Soc* 33(4):228, 1985.

Folstein MF et al: "Mini-Mental State": a practical method for grading the cognitive state of patients for the clinician, *J Psychiatr Res* 12:189, 1975.

Franklin SS et al: Is pulse pressure useful in prediction risk for coronary heart disease? *Circulation* 100:354, 1999.

Frisancho AR: New norms of upper limb fat and muscle areas for assessment of nutritional status, *Am J Clin Nutr* 34:2540, 1981.

Frisancho AR: New standards of weight and body composition by frame size and height for assessment of nutritional status of adults and the elderly, *Am J Clin Nutr* 40:808, 1984.

Gardosi J, Francis A: Controlled trial of fundal height measurement plotted on customized antenatal growth charts, *Br J Obstet Gynecol* 104(4):309-317, 1999.

Goldenring JM, Rosen DS: Getting into adolescent heads: an essential update, *Contemporary Pediatrics*, 21(1):64-90, 2004.

Goldman MP, Fitzpatrick RE: *Cutaneous laser surgery: the art and science of selective photothermolysis,* ed 2, St Louis, 1999, Mosby.

Gotzsche PC, Olsen O: Is screening for breast cancer with mammography justifiable? *Lancet* 355(9198):129-134, 2000.

Grundy S et al: Implications of recent clinical trials for the National Cholesterol Education Program Adult Treatment Panel III Guidelines, *Circulation* 110:227-239, 2004; http://circ.ahajournals.org/ (accessed 12/2005).

Habif TP: *Clinical dermatology,* ed 4, St Louis, 2004, Mosby.

Haller CA, Benowitz NL: Adverse cardiovascular and central nervous system events associated with dietary supplements containing ephedra alkaloids, *N Engl J Med* 343:1833-1842, 2000.

Hardie GE et al: Ethnic descriptors used by African-American and white asthma patients during induced bronchoconstriction, *Chest* 117:935-943, 2000.

Harvey AM et al: *The principles and practice of medicine,* ed 22, Norwalk, CT, Appleton & Lange, 1988.

Hennigan L, Kollar LM, Rosenthal SL: Methods for managing pelvic examination anxiety: individual differences and relaxation techniques, *J Pediatr Health Care* 14(1):9-12, 2000.

Hoberman A, Paradise JL: Acute otitis media: diagnosis and management in the year 2000, *Pediatr Ann* 29(10):609-620, 2000.

Hockenberry MJ: *Wong's essentials of pediatric nursing,* ed 7, St Louis, 2005, Mosby.

Hornor G: Sexual behavior in children: normal or not? *J Pediatr Health Care* Mar-Apr:18(2):57-64, 2004.

Jacobson A: Research for practice: saving limbs with Semmes-Weinstein monofilament, *Am J Nursing* 99(2):76, 1999.

Jacobson RD: Approach to the child with weakness and clumsiness, *Pediatr Clin North Am* 45(1):145-168, 1998.

Jerant AF et al: Early detection and treatment of skin cancer, *Am Fam Physician* 62(2):357-368, 375-376, 381-382, 2000.

Johnson TS, Engstrom JL, Haney SL, Mulcrone SL: Reliability of three length measurement techniques in term infants, *Pediatr Nurs* 25(1):13-17, 1999.

Judge R et al: *Clinical diagnosis,* ed 5, Boston, 1988, Little, Brown.

Kass-Wolff, J, Wilson, E: Pediatric gynecology: assessment strategies and common problems. *Semin Repord Med* 21(4):329-338, 2003.

Kerker BD et al: Identification of violence in the home, *Arch Pediatr Adolesc Med* 154:457-462, 2000.

Kernan WN et al: Phenylpropanolamine and risk of hemorrhagic stroke, *N Engl J Med* 343:1826-1832, 2000.

Khandker RK et al: A decision model and cost-effectiveness analysis of colorectal cancer screening and surveillance guidelines for average-risk adults, *Int J Technol Assess Health Care* 16(3):799-810, 2000.

Knight JR et al: A new brief screen for adolescent substance abuse, *Arch Pediatr Adolesc Med* 153:591-596, 1999.

Knight JR et al: Reliabilities of short substance-abuse screening tests among adolescent medical patients, *Pediatrics* 105:948-953, 2000.

Koop CE: *The Surgeon General's letter on child sexual abuse,* Rockville, Md, 1988, U.S. Department of Health and Human Services.

Kuczmarski MF, Kuczmarski RJ, Najjar M: Descriptive anthropometric reference data for older Americans, *J Am Diet Assoc* 100:59-66, 2000.

Lanham DM et al: Accuracy of tympanic temperature readings in children under 6 years of age, *Pediatr Nurs* 25(1):39-42, 1999.

Lapinsky S: Cardiopulmonary changes in pregnancy: what you need to know, *Women's Health in Primary Care* 2:353, 1999.

Lemmi FO, Lemmi CAE: *Physical assessment findings CD-ROM,* Philadelphia, 2000, WB Saunders.

Levin S et al: *ETHNIC: A framework for culturally competent clinical practice,* 1997.

Lieberman JA III: BATHE: an approach to the interview process in the primary care setting, *J Clin Psychiatry* 58(suppl 3):3-6, 1997.

Lipman TH et al: Assessment of growth by primary health care providers, *J Pediatr Health Care* 14(4):166-171, 2000.

Lowdermilk DL, Perry SE: *Maternity and women's health care,* ed 8, St Louis, 2004, Mosby.

Mattson JE: The language of pain, *Reflections on Nursing Leadership* Fourth quarter:11-14, 2000.

Maynard CK: Differentiate depression from dementia, *The Nurse Practitioner* 28(3):18-27, 2003.

Maugans TA: The SPIRITual history, *Arch Fam Med* 5(1):11-16, 1996.

McCaffery M, Pasero C: Teaching patients to use a numerical pain-rating scale, *Am J Nursing* 99:22, 1999.

McCarty DJ: *Arthritis and allied conditions: a textbook of rheumatology,* ed 2, Philadelphia, 1993, Lea & Febiger.

McClain N et al: Evaluation of sexual abuse in the pediatric patient, *Pediatric Health Care* 14(3):93-102, 2000.

McNeese M: Evaluation of sexual abuse in the pediatric patient, *J Pediatr Health Care* 14(3):93-102, 2000.

Miyasaki-Ching CM: *Chasteen's essentials of clinical dental assisting,* ed 5, St Louis, 1997, Mosby.

Moody CW: Male child sexual abuse, *J Pediatr Health Care* 13:112-119, 1999.

Morrow M: The evaluation of common breast problems, *Am Fam Physician* 61(8):2371-2378, 2385, 2000.

Moyer LA, Mast EE, Altre MJ: Hepatitis C: Part II. Prevention counseling and medical evaluation, *Am Fam Physician* 59(2):349-354, 357, 1999.

National Cholesterol Education Program Expert Panel on Detection, Evaluation, and Treatment of High Blood Cholesterol in Adults: Executive summary of the third report of the National Cholesterol Education Program (NCEP) Expert Panel on Detection, Evaluation, and Treatment of High Blood Cholesterol (Adult Treatment Panel III), *JAMA* 285(19):2486-2497, 2001.

National Institutes of Health: *Report No. 48-4080*, Bethesda, Md, November 1997, The Institutes.

Naway H et al: Concordance of clinical findings and clinical judgment in diagnosis of streptococcal pharyngitis, *Acad Emerg Med* 7(10):1104-1109, 2000.

Nuss R, Manco-Johnson MJ: Venous thrombosus: issues for the pediatrician, *Contemp Pediatr* 17:75, 2000.

Pletcher SD, Goldberg: The diagnosis and treatment of sinusitis. *Advanced Studies in Medicine*, 3(9):495-506, 2003.

Ramsburg KL: Rheumatoid arthritis, *AJN Am J Neuroradiol* 100(11):40-43, 2000.

Rex DK et al: Colorectal cancer prevention 2000: screening recommendations of the American College of Gastroenterology, *Am J Gastroenterol* 95:868-877, 2000.

Rosenthal TC, Puck SM: Screening for genetic risk of breast cancer, *Am Fam Physician* 59(1):99-104, 106, 1999.

Samiy AH, Douglas RG Jr, Barondess JA: *Textbook of diagnostic medicine,* Philadelphia, 1987, Lea & Febiger.

Schulman KA et al: The effects of race and sex on physicians' recommendations for cardiac catheterization, *N Engl J Med* 340:618-626, 1999.

Scott M, Gelhot AR: Gastroesophageal reflux disease: diagnosis and management, *Am Fam Physician* 59(5):1161-1169, 1199, 1999.

Seidel HM et al: *Mosby's guide to physical examination,* ed 6, St Louis, 2006, Mosby.

Sheikh JL, Yesavage JA: Geriatric depression scale: recent evidence and development of a shorter version, *Clin Gerontol* 5:165-172, 1986.

Shinitzky HE, Kub J: The art of motivating behavior change: the use of motivational interviewing to promote health, *Public Health Nurs* 18:178-185, 2001.

Sloan RP et al: Should physicians prescribe religious activities? *N Engl J Med* 342:1913-1916, 2000.

Smith RD, McNamara JJ: The neurological examination of children with school problems, *J Sch Health* 54(7):231-234, 1984.

Sokol RJ, Martier SS, Ager JW: TACE questions: practical prenatal detection of risk-drinking, *Am J Obstet Gynecol* 260(4):863-868, 1989.

Starr NB, Poland C, Dean JA: Malocclusion: How important is that bite? *J Pediatr Health Care* 13:245-247, 1999.

Stuart MR, Lieberman JA III: *The fifteen-minute hour: applied psychotherapy for the primary care physician,* ed 2, New York, 1993, Praeger.

Teoh TG, Fisk NM: Hydramnios, oligohydramnios. In James DK et al, editors: *High-risk pregnancy: management options,* ed 2, Philadelphia, 1999, WB Saunders.

Thibodeau GA, Patton KT: *Anatomy & physiology,* ed 5, St Louis, 2003, Mosby.

Thomas AE et al: A nomogram method for assessing body weight, *Am J Clin Nutr* 29(3):302-304, 1976.

Thompson JM et al: *Mosby's clinical nursing,* ed 4, St Louis, 1997, Mosby.

U.S. Department of Agriculture: MyPyramid, www.mypyramid.gov (accessed 11/2005).

U.S. Department of Health and Human Services: *Clinician's handbook of preventive services,* Washington, DC, 1994, U.S. Government Printing Office.

U.S. Preventive Services Task Force: *Guide to clinical preventive services,* ed 2, Washington, DC, 1996, U.S. Government Printing Office; www.ahrq.gov/clinic/cpsix.htm (accessed 11/2005).

U.S. Preventive Services Task Force: *Guide to clinical preventive services, ed 3: periodic updates,* www.ahrq.gov/clinic/gcpspu.htm (accessed 11/2005).

U.S. Preventive Services Task Force: *Pocket guide to clinical preventive services, 2005,* www.ahrq.gov/clinic/pocketgd.htm (accessed 11/2005).

Varcarolis EM: *Psychiatric nursing clinical guide: assessment tools and diagnosis,* Philadelphia, 1999, WB Saunders.

Videlefsky A et al: Routine vaginal cuff smear testing in post-hysterectomy patients with benign uterine conditions: when is it indicated? *J Am Board Fam Pract* 13(4):233-238, 2000.

Warner PH, Rowe T, Whipple B: Shedding light on the sexual history, *AJN Am J Neuroradiol* 99:34-40, 1999.

Werk LN, Bauchner H, Chessare JB: Medicine for the millennium: demystifying EBM, *Contemp Pediatr* 16:87-107, 1999.

Weston WL, Lane AT, Mortelli JG: *Color textbook of pediatric dermatology,* ed 2, St Louis, 1996, Mosby.

White GM: *Color atlas of regional dermatology,* St Louis, 1994, Mosby.

Whooley MA, Simon GE: Managing depression in medical outpatients, *N Engl J Med* 343:1942-1950, 2000.

Wilson MEH: Keeping quiet, *Arch Pediatr Adolesc Med* 152:1054-1055, 1999.

Wilson SF, Giddens JF: *Health assessment for nursing practice,* ed 3, St Louis, 2005, Mosby.

Wong DL et al: *Whaley and Wong's nursing care of infants and children,* ed 7, St Louis, 2003, Mosby.

Wright RJ: Identification of violence in the community pediatric setting, *Arch Pediatr Adolesc Med* 154:431-433, 2000.

Zitelli BJ, Davis HW: *Atlas of pediatric physical diagnosis,* ed 3, St Louis, 1997, Mosby.

INDEX